Understanding electrocardiography

PHYSIOLOGICAL AND INTERPRETIVE CONCEPTS

UNDERSTANDING
Electrocardiography

PHYSIOLOGICAL AND INTERPRETIVE CONCEPTS

Edwin G. Zalis, M.D., F.A.C.P., F.C.C.P.

Director, Coronary Care Unit, Granada Hills Community Hospital,
Granada Hills; Northridge Hospital, Northridge; Pacoima Memorial
Lutheran Hospital, Lake View Terrace; Serra Memorial Hospital, Sun Valley;
and Clinical Instructor in Medicine, U.C.L.A. School of Medicine,
Los Angeles, California

Mary H. Conover, R.N., B.S.N.Ed.

Instructor in Continuing Education, West Park Hospital, Canoga Park, California,
and Kaiser Hospital, Panorama City, California; Instructor in Electrocardiography
and CCU Nursing, College of the Canyons, Valencia, California,
and California State University, Northridge, California

WITH 341 ILLUSTRATIONS

SAINT LOUIS
The C. V. Mosby Company
1972

W/CB/B 9 8 7 6 5

PREFACE

THE CORONARY CARE UNIT has demonstrated that cautious attention to detecting arrhythmias and various electrocardiographic abnormalities can dramatically improve a patient's chances of surviving an acute myocardial infarction. The key to possibly saving a life is early recognition of unfavorable signs. Therefore the physician must not only have an appreciation of basic electrocardiography but also must rely upon the nurse as a clinical specialist for accurate, early diagnosis and the institution of emergency therapy.

This book is not intended for the specialist in medicine but rather for general practitioners, medical students, nurses, and paramedical personnel. The approach to the subject of electrocardiography is purposely oversimplified, but hopefully it is logical and the coverage comprehensive. Through the use of diagrams and vectors, we have attempted to give the reader a meaningful understanding of the mechanism of arrhythmias. Pattern reading exercises are extensively used.

It is our hope that after studying this book the reader will have achieved at least a modicum of confidence in his ability to understand the electrocardiogram and the oscilloscope monitor.

We gratefully acknowledge the devoted and scholarly assistance of Dr. Sarko M. Tilkian, who reviewed the manuscript in every detail. We are also indebted to the many coronary care nurses throughout the San Fernando Valley who, with care and diligence, collected some of the 178 electrocardiographic tracings that appear in this book. The line drawings were done by William Davis and René Fontan.

Chapter 19 on electrical hazards, an important and often forgotten subject, was written by Edward L. Conover, B.S. (E.E.). We thank him for the generous donation of his time and expertise.

EDWIN G. ZALIS
MARY H. CONOVER

v

CONTENTS

vii

5 Electrical activation of the normal heart, 35

6 Arrhythmias originating in the sinus node, 46

7 Atrial ectopics, 51

8 Ventricular ectopics, 64

Understanding electrocardiography

PHYSIOLOGICAL AND INTERPRETIVE CONCEPTS

1 Anatomy and physiology of the heart

THE HEART AS A PUMP

The four chambers of the heart function as a double pump. The right atrium and ventricle act as one pump to propel the venous blood to the lungs for oxygenation via the pulmonary artery. At the same time, the left atrium and ventricle force the oxygenated blood into the systemic circulation via the aorta (Fig. 1-1).

These two pumps operate simultaneously, although they are completely separate from each other.

SURFACES OF THE HEART

The heart has four surfaces: anterior, posterior, diaphragmatic, and lateral (Fig. 1-2). The anterior and posterior surfaces oppose each other on one plane; the lateral and diaphragmatic surfaces oppose each other on another plane.

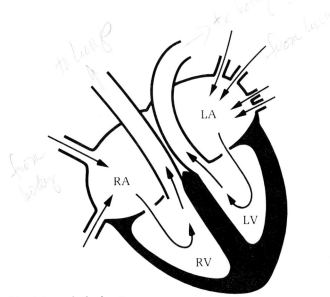

Fig. 1-1. Course of the blood through the heart.

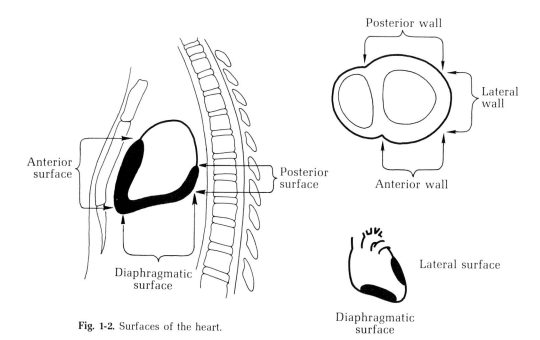

Fig. 1-2. Surfaces of the heart.

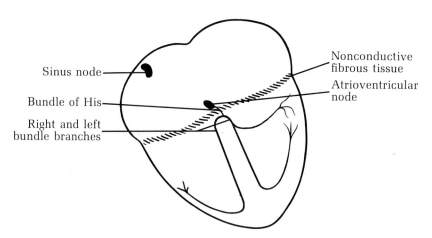

Fig. 1-3. Conductive system of the heart.

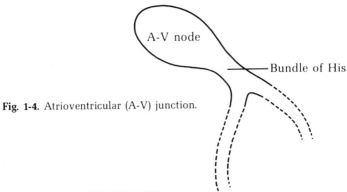

Fig. 1-4. Atrioventricular (A-V) junction.

CONDUCTIVE SYSTEM OF THE HEART

Before the heart can contract, it must be stimulated to do so. Automatically and at regular intervals an electrical current leaves the sinus node, travels through the atria to the atrioventricular node, and then proceeds to the ventricles via the bundle of His. It then invades the ventricular musculature by means of the right and left bundle branches and the Purkinje fibers (Fig. 1-3). Contraction of the heart immediately follows the depolarization of the myocardium.

ATRIOVENTRICULAR (A-V) JUNCTION

A ring of fibrous tissue connects the atria with the ventricles. This tissue will not conduct electrical current. The sole muscular connection between the upper and lower chambers of the heart is the specialized conductive system. We will refer to these structures, rather than to the fibrous ring, as the A-V junction (Fig. 1-4). The A-V junction, then, is composed of the A-V node and the bundle of His with its branches. Normal ventricular activation depends upon an intact and healthy pathway across the A-V junction.

PROPERTIES OF CARDIAC MUSCLE

There are three types of cardiac muscle: atrial, ventricular, and the non-contractile muscle fibers of the conductive system. These muscles have four primary characteristics: excitability, rhythmicity, conductivity, and contractility.

Excitability

The cardiac muscle is electrically irritable due to an ionic imbalance across the membranes of the cells. The degree of negativity within the cell determines its excitability or "responsiveness."

Rhythmicity

In pacemaker cells there is a regular, cyclic fall in potassium conductance during diastole. This causes a threshold to be reached and an action

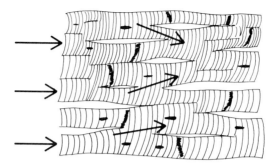

Fig. 1-5. Electrical current spreading along the axis and laterally through the unique interconnections of cardiac muscle.

potential to occur at regular intervals. Thus a current is initiated and propagated along the membranes of all the myocardial cells. This property of cardiac pacemaker cells will be discussed in more detail in Chapter 2.

Conductivity

Conduction velocity is enhanced primarily by the conductive system of the heart that speeds the impulse along at a rate that is six times faster than would be otherwise possible.

The anatomical structure of the heart also influences conduction velocity. Because of a unique interconnection of muscle fibers, the stimulation of one part of the atrium under normal conditions by an impulse that exceeds its threshold produces a response in the entire ventricular muscle mass. If the stimulus is below threshold, none of the cells responds. This phenomenon is called the "all-or-none law."

Fig. 1-5 is a representation of the merging of cells in cardiac muscle. Because of these interconnections, cardiac muscle is said to be syncytial. The electrical current spreads from cell to cell along the axis and laterally through the interconnections more rapidly than in skeletal muscle.

Contractility

The contractility of cardiac muscle is dependent upon many factors, as are the other properties of the myocardium. Two of these factors, the availability of calcium and the integrity of the action potential, will be discussed later in the text. Normally the myocardium contracts in response to each electrical current.

CONDUCTION TIME THROUGH THE HEART

Near the entrance of the superior vena cava is the pacemaker of the heart, the sinus node. The small fibers of the sinus node are continuous with the atrial fibers, so that impulses are spread immediately into the atrial mus-

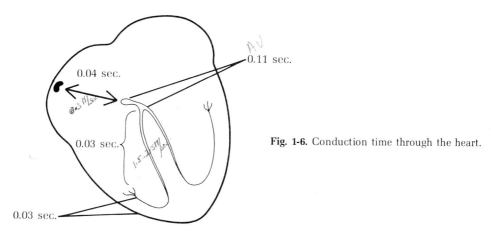

Fig. 1-6. Conduction time through the heart.

culature. The A-V node lies in the lower part of the right atrium, close to the coronary sinus.

Through the use of electrodes within the right ventricle approximate to the bundle of His, exact time values have been recorded for the progress of the current through the A-V junction (Fig. 1-6). There is normally a delay of 0.11 second within the A-V node. This allows the atria to empty their contents into the ventricles before ventricular contraction.

The velocity of conduction through the atria is moderate, about 0.3 meter per second. The impulse reaches the A-V node approximately 0.04 second after it begins in the sinus node. A few specialized Purkinje-like fibers help to speed the impulse conduction directly to the A-V node.

The Purkinje fibers of the ventricles have a transmission velocity of 1.5 to 2.5 meters per second. This is six times faster than can be accomplished by the usual cardiac muscle. It takes approximately 0.03 second for the impulse to traverse the Purkinje system (from the bundle of His to the end of the Purkinje fibers).

When the current leaves the specialized conductive system and flows toward the epicardium, it is again traveling at 0.3 or 0.4 meter per second, the same speed as that achieved in the atrial musculature.

SINUS NODE AS PACEMAKER OF THE HEART

Because the sinus node cycles more rapidly than any other part of the conductive system, it paces the heart. Under abnormal conditions, other parts of the heart may usurp this control by a more rapid cycling or by passively taking over, either because the normal pacemaker has failed or because it is generating its impulses too slowly.

The conductive system has its own intrinsic rate that decreases in rapidity as the pacemaker descends (Fig. 1-7). The A-V node itself has no

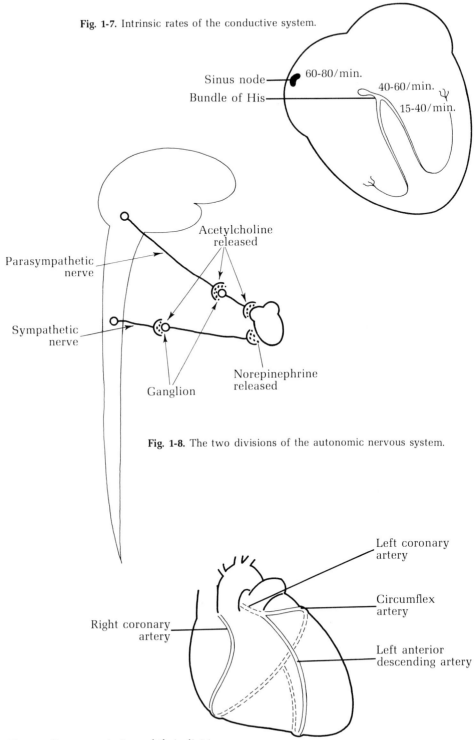

Fig. 1-7. Intrinsic rates of the conductive system.

Sinus node — 60-80/min.

Bundle of His — 40-60/min.

15-40/min.

Acetylcholine released

Parasympathetic nerve

Sympathetic nerve

Norepinephrine released

Ganglion

Fig. 1-8. The two divisions of the autonomic nervous system.

Left coronary artery

Circumflex artery

Right coronary artery

Left anterior descending artery

Fig. 1-9. Coronary arteries and their divisions.

pacemaker cells and hence no power of automaticity. Its chief function is that of delaying the impulse in order to allow for adequate ventricular filling. Therefore in referring to arrhythmias pertaining to this function, the terms "nodal" or "A-V node" will be used. However, the bundle of His has pacemaker cells that will discharge at a rhythmic rate of 40 to 60 times per minute. Because of this, when referring to arrhythmias involving automaticity in the bundle of His, the term "junctional" will be used. Thus we hope to differentiate by simple terms between these two structures and their function within the A-V junction.

Below the bundle of His the Purkinje fibers will discharge at a rate of 15 to 40 times per minute. Normally the sinus node will discharge the other potential pacemakers before self-excitation can occur in them. The sinus node is therefore the pacemaker of the heart.

AUTONOMIC NERVOUS SYSTEM AND CONTROL OF THE HEART

The autonomic nervous system controls the visceral functions of the body. It distributes impulses to the heart, smooth muscle, and glands. The two divisions of the autonomic nervous system are the sympathetic and parasympathetic systems (Fig. 1-8).

Sympathetic nerves

The sympathetic nerves originate in the spinal cord between the first thoracic and second lumbar vertebrae (T-1 and L-2). They supply both the atria and the ventricles, but chiefly the ventricles. Norepinephrine is the mediator, having the effects of increasing the force of cardiac contraction and enhancing the excitability of the heart. It exerts a moderate effect on the atria by increasing the rate of the sinus node.

Parasympathetic nerves

The parasympathetic nerves leave the central nervous system through the cranial and sacral spinal nerves. The vagi are the parasympathetic nerves of the heart (primarily of the atria). Stimulation of the vagi causes the hormone acetylcholine to be released. The effects are supraventricular, causing a slowing of the rate of the sinus node and a decrease in the rate of conduction through the A-V node.

The two divisions of the autonomic nervous system maintain a balance by their opposing influences.

CORONARY CIRCULATION

As the aorta leaves the heart to supply the tissues of the body with blood, its first debt is paid to the heart muscle itself. The right and left coronary arteries arise from within the sinuses of Valsalva (Fig. 1-9).

Right coronary artery

The right coronary artery descends to the right in the atrioventricular groove and turns posteriorly around the inferior margin of the heart. This artery and its branches supply the right ventricle and the diaphragmatic surface of the left ventricle.

Left coronary artery

The left coronary artery divides into the circumflex and the left anterior descending branch. The circumflex artery supplies the lateral wall and the lower half of the posterior wall of the left ventricle. The anterior descending branch supplies the anterior left ventricle and part of the right ventricle.

CORONARY ARTERIES AND THE CONDUCTIVE SYSTEM
Sinus node

In about 55% of hearts a small branch from the right coronary artery supplies the sinus node. A branch from the left circumflex artery supplies the sinus node in the remaining 45%. Occlusion of a coronary artery above the sinus node branch will leave this node ischemic.

A-V node

In 90% of hearts a branch of the distal right coronary artery will supply the A-V node. The left circumflex artery will supply the A-V node in the remaining 10%.

Heart block often complicates a diaphragmatic (inferior) myocardial infarct since occlusion of the right coronary artery may cause not only the infarction but also ischemia of the A-V node.

Bundle of His and its branches

There is an abundant vascular supply to the bundle of His. It receives branches from the A-V nodal artery as well as from the septal branches of the left anterior descending artery.

SUMMARY

The heart is a double pump in which both halves share the same conductive system. Its properties of self-excitation and accelerated conduction differentiate cardiac from skeletal muscle. The heart is under the control of both the sympathetic and parasympathetic nervous systems and receives its blood supply from the right and left coronary arteries and their branches.

STUDY HELPS

1 Draw and label the conductive system of the heart.
2 List and explain the properties of cardiac muscle.
3 What is the purpose of the A-V junction?

4 Where is the normal pacemaker of the heart located? What is it called? Why is it, rather than other parts of the conductive system, the normal pacemaker?

5 Draw the coronary arteries and indicate the blood supply to the sinus node and A-V node.

2 Electrophysiology of the normal heart

INTRODUCTION TO CURRENT FLOW IN THE HEART

The physiological events that precede the mechanical acts of contraction and relaxation are electrochemical in nature. The fluids both inside and outside of the cell membranes of the body are electrolyte solutions made up of positive and negative ions. Current will flow between ions of opposite polarity if they are together within a suitable conductive medium. The current flows from the negative ions to the positive ions in the extracellular fluid.

When the muscle cells of the heart are at rest, the extracellular fluid is mostly positive (Fig. 2-1). Therefore there will be no current flow. But when a muscle cell of the heart is stimulated, there is a change in polarity across the membrane of the cell. A difference then exists between this cell and its neighbor, and a current discharges or flows between the two (Fig. 2-2) until all cells in the same muscle mass have been stimulated to change their polarity.

RESTING MEMBRANE POTENTIAL

Along the inner surface of the resting cell membrane there is an accumulation of an excess number of negative ions (anions). An equal number

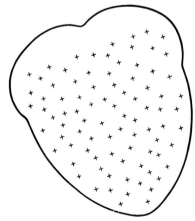

Fig. 2-1. Heart at rest.

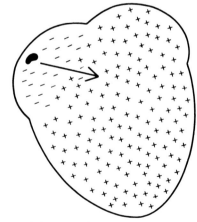

Fig. 2-2. Initiation of current flow within the heart.

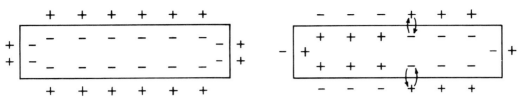

Fig. 2-3. Resting cell.   **Fig. 2-4.** Depolarization.

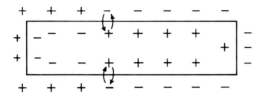

Fig. 2-5. Repolarization.

of positive ions (cations) accumulates outside the membrane. This arrangement of ions of opposite polarity across the membrane results in the development of latent energy in the form of electrical tension. This electrical potential is dependent upon the maintenance of the ionic imbalance and is called the resting membrane potential. The cell is said to be polarized.

DEPOLARIZATION

Fig. 2-3 is a diagrammatic illustration of the polarized muscle cell (the resting cell). There are ions of opposite polarity on either side of the semi-permeable membrane. There is no current flow around the cell since current flows only when negative and positive ions are in the same compartment (the extracellular fluid).

As long as the membrane remains undisturbed, the cell will actively maintain itself in this polarized state. When the rhythmic electrical current arrives from the sinus node, the permeability of the membrane is changed, and the polarity of the cell reverses. This process is called depolarization.

Note that in Fig. 2-4 the permeability of the cell membrane has changed and that the cell is in the process of depolarization. Since now there are both negative and positive ions in the extracellular fluid, a current will flow from negative to positive.

REPOLARIZATION

A fraction of a second after depolarization, the cell will return to its resting state. There will be another reversal of potential, the positive ions again going to the outside of the cell. This process, called repolarization, is shown in Fig. 2-5.

ACTION POTENTIAL

This rapid sequence of events (depolarization and repolarization) is called the action potential. The ionic imbalance across the cell membrane determines the strength of the action potential. This strength in turn determines the speed with which the current is conducted through the muscle mass, so that as the action potential decreases, so does the speed of conduction.

INTEGRITY AND MAINTENANCE OF THE MEMBRANE POTENTIAL

The maintenance of the electrical potential across a cell membrane is dependent upon the integrity of that cell membrane. Injury, ischemia, chemical intoxication, and radical changes in temperature can affect the ability of the membrane to maintain its resting potential.

Apart from these outside forces that may damage the cell, there are other normal forces inherent in the cell. We have said that the resting cell is negative on the inside and positive on the outside. How is it that these negative and positive ions do not equalize each other on either side of the cell membrane?

There are two active forces at work, the sodium pump and the potassium pump. Sodium (Na^+) is pumped to the exterior of the cell. Potassium (K^+) is pumped to the interior of the cell. Also there are negative ions locked within the cell, ions that cannot diffuse across the membrane. These are phosphate, sulfate, and protein ions.

Thus there is a high concentration inside the cell of K^+ and nondiffusable negative ions and a high concentration outside the cell of Na^+. As a result, a membrane potential develops. "Potential" means power that exists and is ready for action. The action potential occurs when the sodium permeability of the membrane is changed and the Na^+ rushes to the interior of the cell, causing a reversal of polarity (depolarization). K^+ rapidly leaves the cell, initiating repolarization, and the cell returns quickly to its resting state.

INITIATION OF IMPULSES WITHIN THE SINUS NODE

The pacemaker cells have a slightly different physiology than their sister cells in the myocardium. They are capable of self-excitation. In atrial and ventricular cells the inward and outward currents balance each other to maintain a constant resting membrane potential. In the cells of the sinus node a constant resting membrane potential is not maintained. Rather, there is a slow diastolic depolarization (the cell becomes more positive on the inside) until the threshold is reached and the action potential occurs, marked by a sudden and rapid influx of Na^+ into the cell. This slow diastolic depolarization is thought to be due to a fall in K^+ conductance. That is, K^+ does not leave the cell. This, combined with the passive diffusion of Na^+ into the cell, means that the pacemaker cell becomes more and more positive intracellularly until eventually a threshold is reached (self-excitation). The

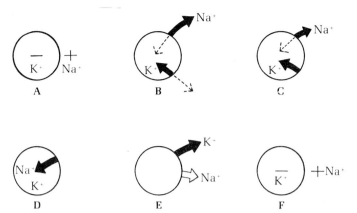

Fig. 2-6. A, Cell at rest. **B,** Ionic pumps and membrane conductance maintain resting membrane potential. **C,** Decay of potassium (K⁺) conductance causes slow diastolic depolarization. **D,** Depolarization. A threshold is reached and sodium (Na⁺) rushes in. The sodium pump is inactive. **E,** Potassium rapidly leaves the cell to bring about the beginning of repolarization. **F,** The cell returns to its resting state.

subsequent rapid exchange of ions across the cell membrane (depolarization) is propagated through the myocardium. The cell returns quickly to its resting state, mainly due to a rapid exit of K⁺ from the cell. The cycle then begins again, the cycle length being directly dependent upon the rate at which K⁺ conductance falls. These events are diagrammatically illustrated in Fig. 2-6.

REFRACTORY PERIODS
The single cell

The individual muscle cell must return to its resting state before it is ready or able to depolarize again. Repolarization must be complete before the cell can accept another stimulus. If it is stimulated during the process of repolarization, before it has regained its resting state, it will reject or *refract* the stimulus. This is termed the refractory period.

The heart as a whole

Because the heart is made up of many individual cells, each with its own particular depolarization and repolarization process, there will be nonrefractory and refractory cells present simultaneously in the heart.

When depolarization has just been completed, all cells are refractory and unable to accept a stimulus. This is called the *absolute* refractory period (Fig. 2-7).

The *relative* refractory period, or vulnerable period, of the heart occurs when some cells are polarized (positive) and others are still depolarized (negative) (Fig. 2-8). The polarized cells are nonrefractory and are therefore able to accept a stimulus. The depolarized cells are still refractory. A strong

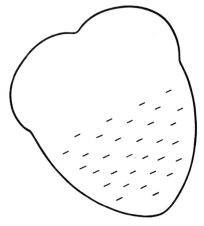

Fig. 2-7. Absolute refractory period of the heart.

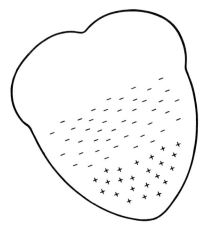

Fig. 2-8. Relative refractory period of the heart.

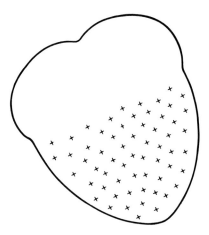

Fig. 2-9. Nonrefractory period of the heart.

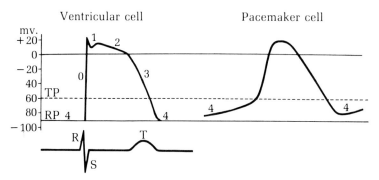

Fig. 2-10. Action potential. TP = Threshold potential. RP = Resting potential.

stimulus to the heart at this time may result in electrical chaos, hence the term "vulnerable."

The completely repolarized heart is ready to adequately and efficiently respond to another stimulus and is thus called nonrefractory (Fig. 2-9).

PHASES OF THE ACTION POTENTIAL

By using microelectrodes it is possible to record the sequence of electrical potentials within a cardiac muscle cell during the process of depolarization and repolarization (Fig. 2-10).

Phase 0

The rapid upstroke of the action potential represents the depolarization of the cell. It extends from the threshold potential (TP) to the peak of the action potential. Na^+, which in the resting state is more abundant in the extracellular fluid, suddenly and rapidly rushes into the cell when a threshold is reached. This causes a sudden reversal of potential (the cell that was negative on the inside is now positive) and produces the spike of the action potential.

Phase 1

Phase 1 is the initial stage of repolarization. It has a sudden, brief beginning.

Phase 2

During approximately the next 0.1 second the repolarization process slows down, causing a plateau in the action potential. This plateau, which does not occur in skeletal muscle, allows the cardiac muscle a more sustained contraction. (The strength and duration of the muscle contraction are directly proportional to the amplitude and duration of the action potential.)

Phase 3

There is then a sudden acceleration of the rate of repolarization as K^+ leaves the cell in response to the influx of Na^+.

Phase 4

The beginning of phase 4 represents the resting potential (RP) of the cell. Repolarization has been completed, Na^+ has been actively pumped back out of the cell, and K^+ has been taken back in. This phase extends from the beginning of the resting potential to the threshold potential (diastole).

In Fig. 2-10 you will notice that the slope of phase 4 is steeper in the pacemaker cell. This is because of a time-dependent decay in potassium conductance. This, combined with a passive diffusion of sodium back into the cell, causes a threshold to be reached. Depolarization is thus self-initiated in the pacemaker cells. This buildup of positive ions is more rapid in the sinus node, which discharges the lower pacemakers before they have a chance to discharge themselves. The atrial and ventricular cells reach phase 0 abruptly since they are dependent upon the pacemaker cells for their depolarization.

MEMBRANE RESPONSIVENESS

The term "membrane responsiveness" refers to the relationship of the resting membrane potential at excitation to the rate of depolarization during phase 0 of the action potential (the rising phase). Conduction velocity and the ability of the cardiac muscle fiber to respond to a stimulus will be affected if these factors are changed.

The normal resting membrane potential is usually -85 to -90 millivolts (mv.). The higher the level of this membrane potential (the more negativity within the cell), the quicker will be the rate of depolarization during phase 0 and the higher will be the amplitude of the action potential. Conversely, as the level of the membrane potential (voltage) is lowered, so is the rate of depolarization during phase 0 and so is the height of the action potential. Since conduction velocity is directly dependent upon these two factors, conduction is also slowed. At about -70 mv., conduction disturbance will begin to appear. Complete block and lack of response will appear at about -55 mv.

Many of the antiarrhythmic agents will affect membrane responsiveness by their ability to change either the level of the threshold potential or the duration of the action potential. A change in either of these mechanisms will affect the duration of the absolute refractory period.

VECTORS

A vector is a symbolic representation of a physical force having both direction and magnitude. A current will flow from negative (depolarized) tissue to positive (polarized) tissue. This current flow is symbolized by an arrow (vector). The length of the arrow indicates the size (amplitude) of the vector force (the strength of the current). The point of the arrow indicates the direction of current flow, which is always from negative tissue to positive tissue.

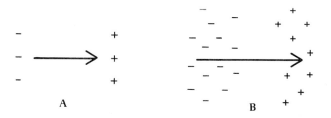

Fig. 2-11. **A,** Few cells and a small vector. **B,** Many cells and a large vector.

In vector *A* of Fig. 2-11 there are only a few negative and positive charges. This represents a thin muscle with few cells and therefore a small current. There is only a slight electrical potential between these two areas. Therefore the vector is short.

Vector *B* represents a thicker muscle mass with more cells. There is a greater number of negative and positive charges. Therefore the current will be greater. A longer vector is drawn to indicate this greater electrical potential between the two areas. Notice that in both examples the current flows from a negative area to a positive area.

Briefly, then:

1   The length of each vector indicates the strength of the electrical potential between the negative and positive areas.
2   This potential in turn depends upon the total amount of polarization and depolarization present.
3   The direction of current flow is indicated by an arrow.
4   The point of the arrow represents the positive end of the vector.
5   The length of the arrow represents the strength of the current.

The atrial vector, which represents the current generated during atrial depolarization, is relatively small since fewer cells are involved (Fig. 2-12, *A*). The ventricular vector is much larger since it represents the depolarization of the thick ventricular muscle mass (Fig. 2-12, *B*).

ELECTRICAL AXIS OF THE HEART

In the normal heart, current flows primarily from the base to the apex. It flows from the depolarized (negative) cells to the polarized (positive) cells.

This preponderant direction of current flow in the heart is known as the axis. It is expressed only as a direction, not as a magnitude (Fig. 2-13).

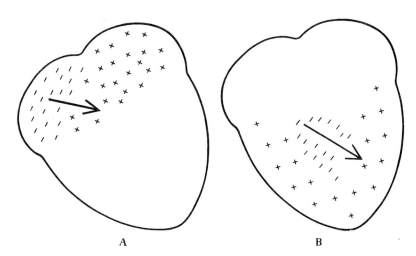

Fig. 2-12, A, Atrial vector. **B,** Ventricular vector.

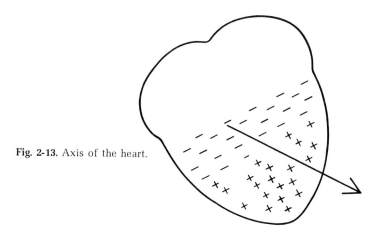

Fig. 2-13. Axis of the heart.

SUMMARY

Myocardial depolarization is possible because of an ionic imbalance across the cell membranes. The resting membrane potential is dependent upon this ionic imbalance and determines the rate of rise and amplitude of the action potential, which in turn determines conduction velocity. Depolarization and repolarization are two divisions of the action potential; depolarization represents a reversal potential (exchange of ions), and repolarization represents a return to the original potential (another exchange of ions). This is a cyclic process in pacemaker cells because of the quicker fall in potassium conductance and the lower resistance to sodium influx that trigger the depolarization process. The pacemaker cells of the sinus node cycle faster than other pacemaker cells, so that the sinus node dominates the heart.

An action potential reached in one cell of the myocardium is propagated to all myocardial cells. This propagation (or flow) is a current or vector that is cyclic according to heart rate and is usually identical in direction and magnitude each time. The axis of the heart is the main direction that this current takes.

The refractory period of the heart occurs during the action potential, the absolute refractory period occurs during depolarization, and the relative refractory period occurs during repolarization.

STUDY HELPS

1 Explain the interrelationships of stimulation, depolarization, and contraction.
2 How is it possible for electrical currents to flow within the muscles and organs of the body?
3 Differentiate between axis and vector.
4 In what direction does current flow relative to tissue polarity?
5 Explain the relative and absolute refractory periods. Explain each as it pertains to a single cell and to the heart as a whole.

3 Recording equipment

INTRODUCTION

The electrocardiogram (ECG) is a graphic recording of the electrical potentials rhythmically produced by the heart muscle.

The heart is unique in that it contracts automatically and rhythmically due to electrical impulses generated within a remarkable conduction system. These impulses result in the production of weak electrical currents that diffuse throughout the body, which acts as a volume conductor. Electrodes are applied to the surface of the body and connected to an electrocardiographic apparatus, which is basically a galvanometer. These electrical currents are then passed through an amplifier and accurately recorded. This recording is called an ECG. It will faithfully indicate the strength of the current and the direction in which it is flowing.

The ECG provides information that is useful in a variety of clinical situations, including the following:

1 Arrhythmias
2 Atrial and ventricular hypertrophy
3 Myocardial infarction
4 Pericarditis
5 Systemic diseases that affect the heart
6 Effect of cardiac drugs, especially digitalis and quinidine
7 Electrolyte and metabolic disturbances

EQUIPMENT
Strip recorder

When it is combined with an amplifier, the strip recorder will give a permanent record of the electrical potentials of the cardiac cycle. The record is produced by the movements of a heated stylus on the wax-coated ECG paper. A three-channel cardiograph (Fig. 3-1) will automatically record all twelve ECG leads in 10 seconds.

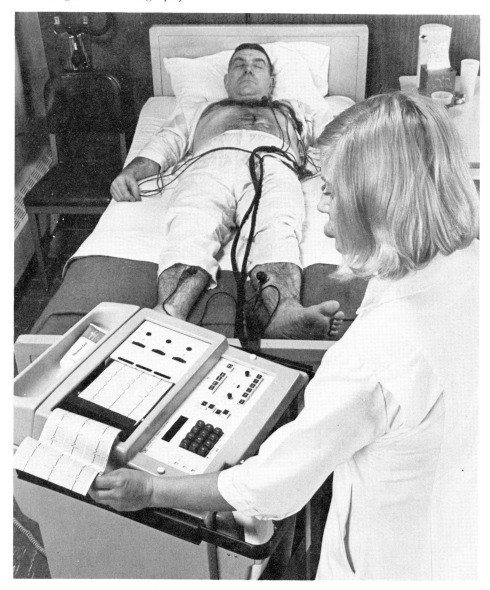

Fig. 3-1. Strip recorder. (Courtesy Hewlett-Packard, Palo Alto, Calif.)

Computer concept

ECG signals may be transmitted over telephone lines or via magnetic tape to a computer system that automatically prints out measurements and interpretive statements (Fig. 3-2). These printouts will assist the physician in his diagnosis.

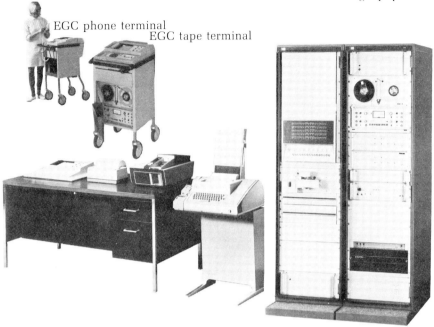

EGC phone terminal
EGC tape terminal

Fig. 3-2. Computerized ECG interpretive system. (Courtesy Hewlett-Packard, Palo Alto, Calif.)

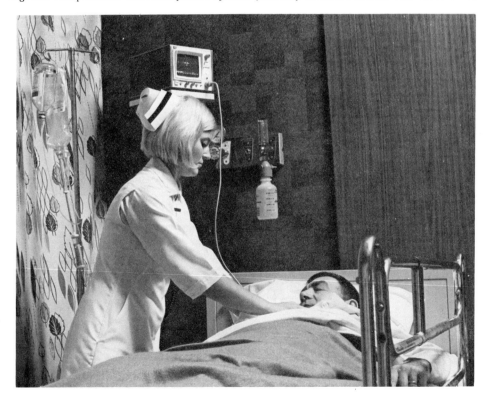

Fig. 3-3. Oscilloscope. (Courtesy Hewlett-Packard, Palo Alto, Calif.)

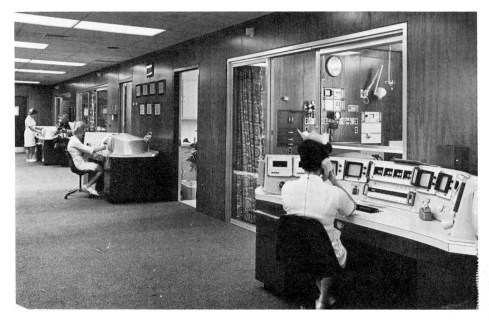

Fig. 3-4. Central station patient monitors. (Courtesy Hewlett-Packard, Palo Alto, Calif.)

Oscilloscope

The patient monitor, or oscilloscope (Fig. 3-3), displays the electrical events of the heart in a continuous pattern on a fluorescent screen. The oscilloscope does not give a permanent record unless it is combined with the strip recorder. It is of particular value in the constant monitoring of patients with either myocardial infarction or serious arrhythmias. For monitoring in the coronary care unit, the electrodes are usually placed on the chest. A cable connects these electrodes to the oscilloscope.

It is possible to display the ECG, pulse, or arterial pressure wave forms and derive the heart rate from any one of these. The heart rate may then be displayed on a bar graph on the same monitor.

Central station patient monitors

ECG wave forms that are being recorded at patients' bedsides are transmitted to a central station (Fig. 3-4), where it is possible for a nurse to observe several ECGs at once.

Computerized patient-monitoring system

The computerized patient-monitoring system (Fig. 3-5) continually monitors, stores, and retrieves information on command, so that the patient's past and present physiological parameters are immediately available to the physician for his evaluation.

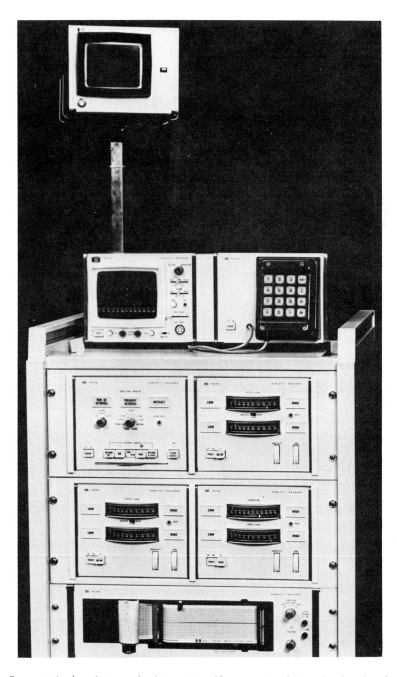

Fig. 3-5. Computerized patient-monitoring system. (Courtesy Hewlett-Packard, Palo Alto, Calif.)

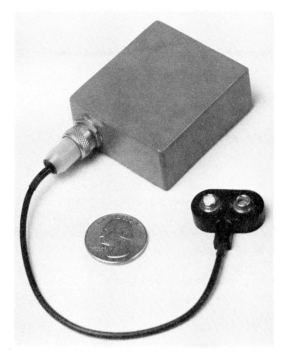

Fig. 3-6. Battery for monitoring by telemetry.

Telemetry

A small, lightweight, battery-powered transmitter worn in a belt allows a patient to ambulate while being monitored (Fig. 3-6). The cable from the electrodes is attached to this transmitter. The signal is then relayed to the central station oscilloscope, where it is amplified and displayed. Since telemetry is battery powered, the hazards with electrical shock have been virtually eliminated.

4 The lead systems

A LEAD AND ITS AXIS DEFINED

A bipolar lead is composed of two electrodes, one positive and one negative. An imaginary line drawn between these two electrodes is known as the axis of the lead.

ELECTROCARDIOGRAPHY AND ITS FUNCTIONS

The heart is an electrical field in which currents flow in repetitive patterns according to the heart rate. These currents can be detected at the level of the skin by the use of two electrodes of opposite polarity that are placed at opposite poles of the electrical field. The electrodes are attached to an amplifier within an oscilloscope or strip recorder. These instruments will then accurately record the electrical events of the heart, namely direction of current flow and magnitude of the current. The interpretation of these events is the basis for the electrocardiographic diagnosis of arrhythmias and cardiac disease.

Direction of current flow

Direction of current flow will be indicated in the following manner. A current flowing toward the positive terminal of the lead axis will be recorded as a positive (upright) deflection. A current directed toward the negative terminal of the lead axis will be recorded as a negative (downward) deflection. A current directed exactly perpendicular to the lead axis will record a net zero potential because both electrodes will sense exactly the same force. This will be indicated by either a straight (isoelectric) line or a deflection that is equal in both directions.

Magnitude of current

The strength of the vector will be indicated by the recording of a small deflection for a weak vector and a large deflection for a strong vector.

BIPOLAR AND UNIPOLAR LEADS

The bipolar leads compare the electrical potentials between two electrode (− and +) terminals. The axis of the lead is determined by the two electrodes. The ECG from a bipolar lead will be a reflection of the orientation of the cardiac vectors to this axis. In the twelve-lead ECG only three of the leads are bipolar. They are leads I, II, and III.

The unipolar leads determine the electrical potentials at a single lead site, relatively uninfluenced by a reference to another electrode. The axis of the unipolar lead is an imaginary line drawn from the positive exploring electrode to the center of the heart (zero potential).

THE THREE STANDARD LIMB LEADS

The arms and legs are linear extensions of the electrical field surrounding the heart. Therefore an electrode placed on the right arm would sense the same electrical potentials that would be sensed at the right shoulder. The same would apply to electrodes on the other extremities. With this in mind, it is easier to appreciate that the axes of the three bipolar limb leads form a triangle around the heart. This is known as *Einthoven's triangle* and is shown in Fig. 4-1.

The axis of lead I extends from shoulder to shoulder. The negative electrode is on the right arm, and the positive electrode is on the left arm.

The axis of lead II extends from the right shoulder to the left leg or to a point just below the rib cage. The negative electrode is on the right arm, and the positive electrode is on the left leg.

The axis of lead III extends from the left shoulder to the left leg or to

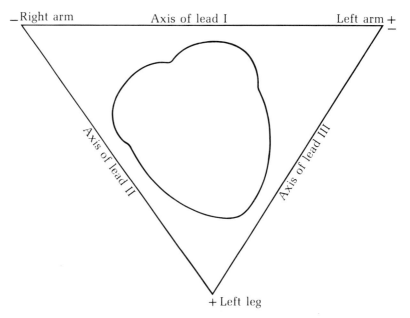

Fig. 4-1. Axes of the three standard limb leads form Einthoven's triangle.

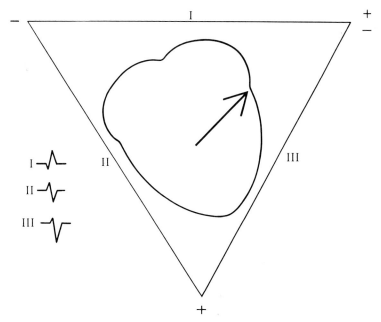

Fig. 4-2. Cardiac vector related to the three standard limb leads.

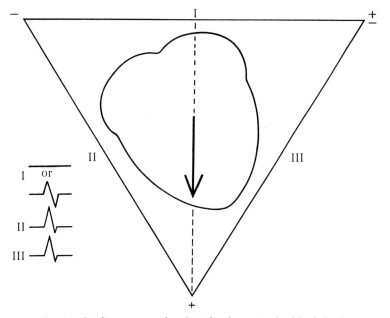

Fig. 4-3. Cardiac vector related to the three standard limb leads.

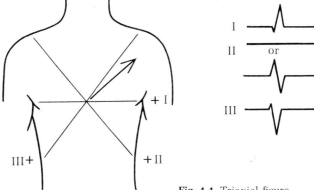

Fig. 4-4. Triaxial figure.

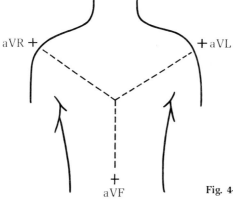

Fig. 4-5. Axes of the unipolar limb leads.

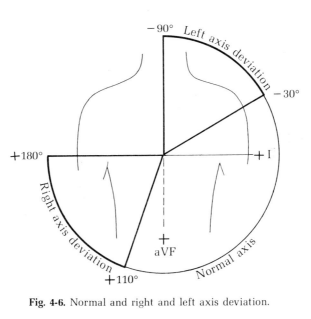

Fig. 4-6. Normal and right and left axis deviation.

a point just below the rib cage. The negative electrode is on the left arm, and the positive electrode is on the left leg.

The sum of the potentials of these three leads is zero, and if plotted, will be found to be at the center of the triangle.

CARDIAC VECTORS RELATED TO THE LEAD AXIS

The vector in Fig. 4-2 would cause a positive deflection to be written in lead I because the flow is toward the positive terminal of the lead axis.

The polarity of the deflection in leads II and III would be negative since the current is directed toward the negative terminal of the lead axis.

The vector in Fig. 4-3 is exactly perpendicular to the axis of lead I, which will reflect no electrical potential at all. In this lead each electrode senses the same amount of current; therefore a flat line or a complex with equal positive and negative deflections will be written. Leads II and III will have a strong positive deflection since the vector is directed toward the positive terminal.

THE TRIAXIAL FIGURE

Perhaps the relationship of the vectors to Einthoven's triangle can be more easily seen if the three axes are shifted so that they all pass through what is considered the zero point of the heart's electrical field.

The arrow in Fig. 4-4 represents the mean ventricular vector. The relationship of the vector to each lead axis is easily seen. The vector is perpendicular to the axis of lead II, causing equal deflections on either side of the isoelectric line. In lead I the current flow is directed toward the positive terminal, producing a positive deflection. In lead III the current flows toward the negative terminal, producing a negative deflection.

AUGMENTED LEADS (UNIPOLAR EXTREMITY LEADS)

There are three unipolar extremity leads, aV_R, aV_L, and aV_F (Fig. 4-5). The letter "a" stands for augmented, a term that was added when it was discovered that by eliminating a negative electrode the amplitude of the recording was augmented by 50%. "V" means vector. The inferior capital letters "R," "L," and "F" indicate where the positive electrode is placed—the right arm, left arm, and left leg (foot).

The unipolar lead compares the electrical potentials of the heart with zero. This zero potential represents the electrical potentials at the center of the heart. The axis of the lead is an imaginary line drawn from the lead site to the center of the heart.

NORMAL AXIS OF THE HEART

Since each unipolar limb lead is perpendicular to a bipolar standard lead axis, we have a useful reference for plotting the cardiac vector.

The normal axis lies between +110 and −30 degrees, or just beyond the quadrant described by the axes of aV$_F$ and lead I (Fig. 4-6). A mean ventricular vector beyond these borders would be considered a marked axis deviation.

LEFT AXIS DEVIATION

A deviation of the mean QRS vector of between −30 and −90 degrees to the left is considered abnormal (Fig. 4-6).

The cardiac vector in Fig. 4-7 is directed abnormally to the left and toward the positive terminal of lead I, causing a positive deflection. The aV$_F$ electrode senses a current flowing away from it. Therefore a negative deflection is written.

The cardiac vector in Fig. 4-8 represents an extreme left axis deviation. The vector is perpendicular to the axis of lead I, causing a flat line or an equiphasic deflection (the positive and negative electrodes sense the same electrical force). The vector is directed away from the positive electrode of aV$_F$; therefore a strong negative deflection is recorded.

RIGHT AXIS DEVIATION

When the mean QRS vector is deviated to the right between +110 and +180 degrees, it is considered abnormal (Fig. 4-6).

The cardiac vector in Fig. 4-9 is directed abnormally to the right and toward the negative half of the lead I axis, causing a negative deflection to be recorded. The aV$_F$ electrode senses a vector coming toward it; therefore, a positive deflection is written.

The cardiac vector in Fig. 4-10 represents an extreme right axis deviation. The vector is flowing directly toward the negative terminal of lead I; therefore a negative deflection is written. The aV$_F$ electrode senses a vector perpendicular to its axis; therefore a flat line or a deflection that is equal in each direction is written.

PRECORDIAL LEADS

The chest (precordial) leads are unipolar. That is, each lead consists of one positive electrode and a zero potential reference point. This zero potential is the center of the heart. The axis of these leads is an imaginary line drawn from the positive electrode to the heart center.

Axis of V$_1$

The positive electrode of V$_1$ is placed at the fourth intercostal space of the right sternal border. The axis extends from this site to the heart center, as seen in Fig. 4-11.

An electrical force flowing toward the electrode of the lead would cause a positive deflection. If the current flows perpendicular to the axis, equal pos-

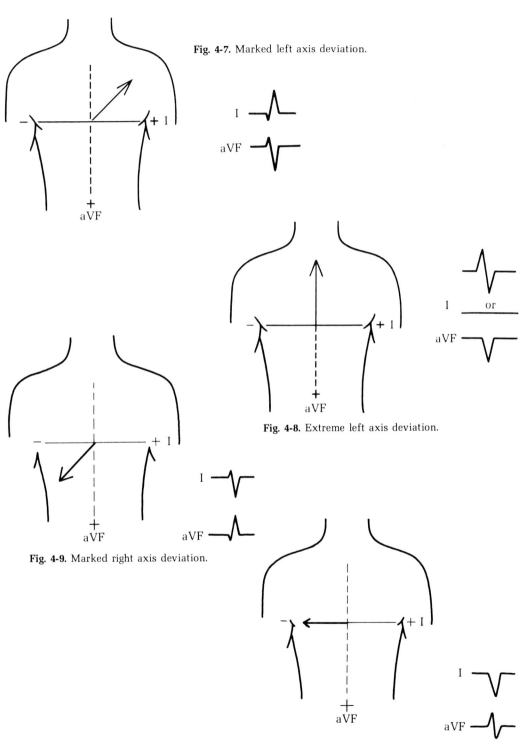

Fig. 4-7. Marked left axis deviation.

Fig. 4-8. Extreme left axis deviation.

Fig. 4-9. Marked right axis deviation.

Fig. 4-10. Extreme right axis deviation.

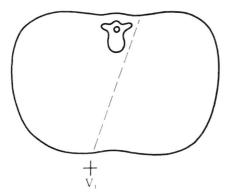

Fig. 4-11. Axis of lead V_1.

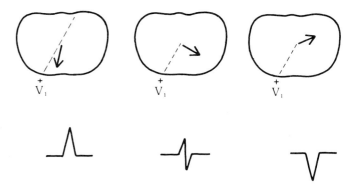

Fig. 4-12. Cardiac vector related to the axis of V_1.

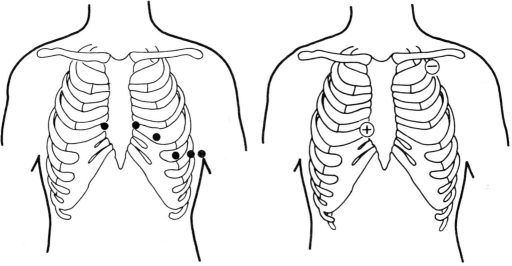

Fig. 4-13. Precordial lead sites.

Fig. 4-14. MCL.

itive and negative deflections will be recorded. A negative deflection is recorded if the current flows away from the electrode, as seen in Fig. 4-12.

Precordial lead sites

The precordial lead sites (Fig. 4-13) are as follows:

V_1 Fourth intercostal space, right sternal border
V_2 Fourth intercostal space, left sternal border
V_3 Equidistant between V_2 and V_4
V_4 Fifth intercostal space, left midclavicular line
V_5 Lateral to V_4 at the anterior axillary line
V_6 Lateral to V_5 at the midaxillary line

MCL

A selective modified chest electrode (MCL) is useful for monitoring in the coronary care unit (Fig. 4-14). It is a bipolar lead that simulates the unipolar precordial lead, V_1. The positive electrode is placed as is the electrode for V_1, on the right side of the sternum between the fourth and fifth intercostal spaces. The negative electrode is placed just below the left midclavicle.

HIS BUNDLE ELECTROGRAM

Because the conventional twelve-lead ECG yields indirect information about the activity of the A-V junction during the cardiac cycle, only inferences can be made regarding atrioventricular and intraventricular conduction time. The catheter technique of His bundle recordings has therefore been a significant advance in the understanding of the mechanism of arrhythmias.

His bundle electrogram (HBE) is the term given to the bipolar lead that records the electrical activity of the A-V junction. The catheter is introduced through the femoral vein and advanced into the right ventricle just .next to the bundle of His and right bundle branch.

The HBE lead will not record left bundle branch events since the catheter is in the right ventricle. There are three deflections: atrial (A), bundle of His (H), and ventricular (V). The measurable intervals, then, would be the atrio-His (A-H) and His-ventricular (H-V) intervals.

The advantages of such a recording will become increasingly apparent as you become more familiar with the arrhythmias. For now, let it suffice to say that with the HBE one of the "silent zones" of the ECG is no longer silent. Thus we have a more meaningful knowledge of the electrodynamics of cardiac arrhythmias.

SUMMARY

There are unipolar and bipolar leads. The unipolar leads compare the electrical potentials at a particular lead site with the zero potential at the heart center. The bipolar leads compare the electrical potentials between two lead sites, a negative electrode and a positive electrode.

The cardiac vectors sensed through these leads are recorded according to the magnitude and direction of current flow. This recording is called an ECG.

STUDY HELPS

1 Explain what is meant by the axis of a lead.
2 What information is given by the ECG?
3 How does a bipolar lead differ from a unipolar lead?
4 Draw Einthoven's triangle and a cardiac vector. Draw the ECG tracing that reflects this particular vector in each of the three standard leads.

5 Electrical activation of the normal heart

CONFIGURATION OF THE NORMAL ECG

The normal ECG is composed of a P wave, a QRS complex, and a T wave (Fig. 5-1).

P WAVE

The P wave represents the depolarization of the atria. The duration of the P wave (not over 0.10 second in the normal person) indicates the time it takes for the depolarization current to pass through the atrial musculature. Because the atria are thin-walled structures, a small deflection will be written. Furthermore, since the P vector is traveling in a leftward and inferior direction, the current will flow toward the positive terminals of leads I, II, aV$_F$, aV$_L$ and V$_3$ to V$_6$. A positive deflection will therefore be written in these leads (Fig. 5-2).

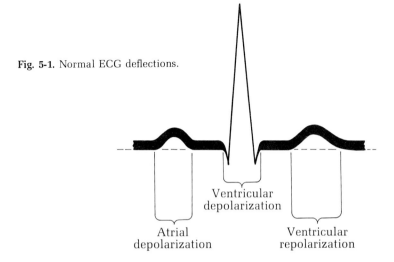

Fig. 5-1. Normal ECG deflections.

Ventricular depolarization

Atrial depolarization

Ventricular repolarization

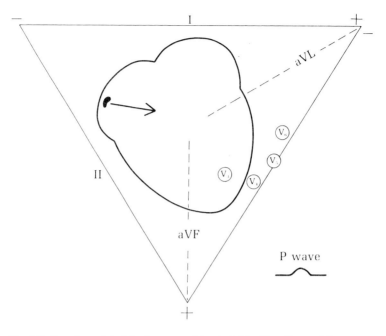

Fig. 5-2. P vector related to the axes of leads I, II, aV_F, aV_L, and V_3 to V_6.

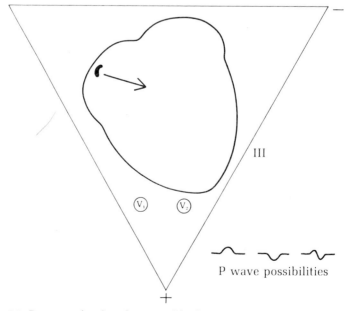

Fig. 5-3. P vector related to the axes of leads III, V_1, and V_2.

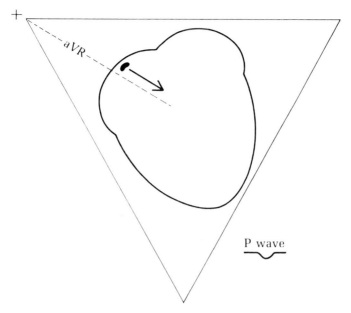

Fig. 5-4. P vector related to the axis of lead aV_R.

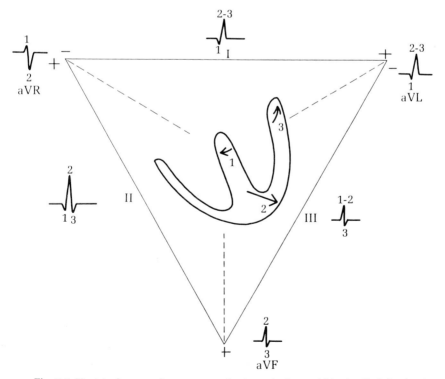

Fig. 5-5. Ventricular complexes as seen in the unipolar and bipolar limb leads.

Depending upon the position of the heart in the body and upon the orientation of the atrial vector to the positive terminals, the P wave may be upright, diphasic, flat, or inverted in leads III, V_1, and V_2 (Fig. 5-3).

The P wave is normally inverted in lead aV_R because the P vector travels away from this electrode (Fig. 5-4).

VENTRICULAR COMPLEX

The shape of the ventricular complex is determined by the orientation of the vectors to the lead axis.

Ventricular complex as seen in the unipolar and bipolar extremity leads

1 The interventricular (I-V) septum is the first ventricular structure to depolarize. The current moves from left to right.
2 The ventricular muscle mass is the next to depolarize. Since the left ventricle is thicker than the right ventricle, it is this strong vector that is sensed by all of the leads.
3 The epicardial surface at the base of the heart is the last to depolarize, causing a small vector to flow toward the base of the heart (Fig. 5-5).

Ventricular complex as seen in the precordial leads

Since the left ventricular activation produces a stronger vector, the leads over the right ventricle (V_1 and V_2) will record left ventricular depolarization rather than the weaker vector generated by the right ventricle (Fig. 5-6). Since the stronger current is flowing away from the positive electrode, a negative deflection will be written in these leads (S wave).

As the precordial electrodes are placed closer to the left ventricle, the greater electrical current generated by this ventricle flows more and more toward the positive electrode and is sensed more strongly. Thus the R wave can be seen to become progressively larger (V_3 to V_6). In other words, the size of the R wave increases in proportion to the proximity of the precordial electrode to the left ventricle. This phenomenon is called "R wave progression."

T WAVE

The T wave is the result of the repolarization process in the ventricle and indicates what is referred to as the vulnerable period. At this time the ventricles are in a relative refractory condition, and a stimulus during the T wave may precipitate a serious ventricular arrhythmia (Fig. 5-7).

Electrophysiology

Contrary to expectation, the first ventricular area to depolarize (the I-V septum) is not the first part to repolarize. If it were, a negative T wave would often be inscribed. Rather, the epicardium is the first to repolarize.

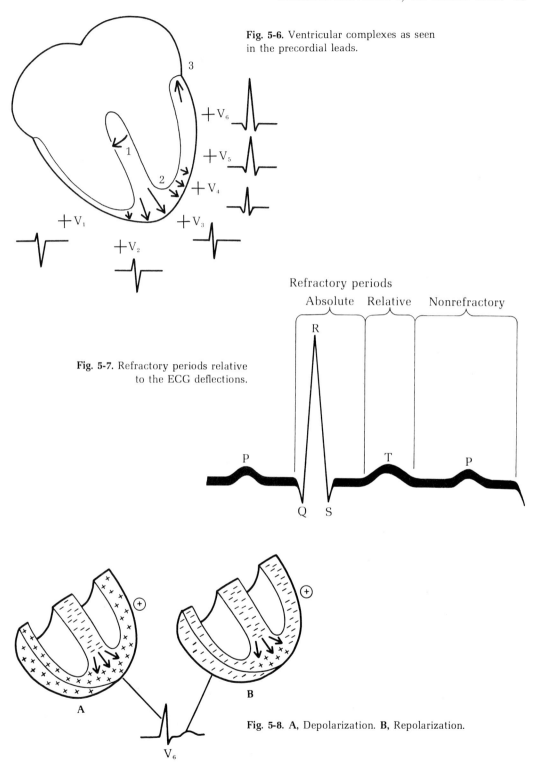

Fig. 5-6. Ventricular complexes as seen in the precordial leads.

Fig. 5-7. Refractory periods relative to the ECG deflections.

Refractory periods

Absolute   Relative   Nonrefractory

Fig. 5-8. A, Depolarization. **B,** Repolarization.

This is thought to occur because the endocardium recovers more slowly than the epicardium due to the pressures of contraction and reduction in coronary blood flow. The repolarization process, then, passes from epicardium to endocardium.

In Fig. 5-8 it can be seen that the depolarization process passes from endocardium to epicardium and that the current is also oriented in this direction (from negative to positive). Although the repolarization process proceeds in the opposite direction (from epicardium to endocardium), the *current still flows from negative to positive*. The vector is therefore oriented toward the positive electrode, causing a positive T wave to be inscribed.

Factors changing the sequence of repolarization

Anything that changes normal repolarization as described will also change the T wave.

Slow conduction resulting from bundle branch block, ventricular extrasystoles, or ventricular hypertrophy may cause a change in the polarity of the T wave. These conditions change the direction of the depolarization current (mean electrical axis) and thus influence the repolarization process. For example, in left bundle branch block the right ventricle begins to repolarize before the left ventricle, producing a T wave that is of opposite polarity to the QRS.

Prolonged periods of depolarization in portions of the ventricle will also change the sequence of repolarization. Ischemia, whether acute, chronic, or associated with coronary occlusion, is the most common cause of increased periods of depolarization. In the presence of ischemia the period of depolarization increases disproportionately.

For example, if there is prolonged depolarization in the apex, it is unable to repolarize first as is normal. The base of the heart will therefore repolarize first, causing a vector in the direction opposite to the normal.

Effect of toxic conditions

Even the slightest change in the period of depolarization of only one portion of the ventricles can cause T wave changes. T wave abnormalities are sensitive indicators of a variety of conditions, including acid-base imbalance, metabolic diseases, hyperventilation, autonomic hyperactivity, and the effects of various drugs.

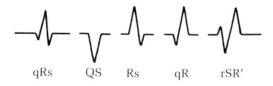

qRs   QS   Rs   qR   rSR′

Fig. 5-9. QRS deflections.

DEFINITION OF QRS DEFLECTIONS

Since the deflections of the ECG are the result of cardiac vectors and their relationship to the axes of the leads, the QRS complex will normally be shaped differently in the various leads. Each lead represents a view of the heart from another angle.

In Fig. 5-9 a base line may be seen to run through the length of the ECG tracing. This is known as the *isoelectric* line. It is present whenever there is no current flowing in the heart, that is, when the heart is either all negative after depolarization or all positive after repolarization.

A deflection above the line is a positive deflection. A deflection below the line is a negative deflection. All positive deflections are R waves. If there is more than one positive deflection, the second one will be called R′ (R prime). A negative deflection before the R wave is a Q wave. A negative deflection that occurs after the R wave is an S wave. Sometimes there is no positive deflection at all. The sole negative deflection would be called a QS complex.

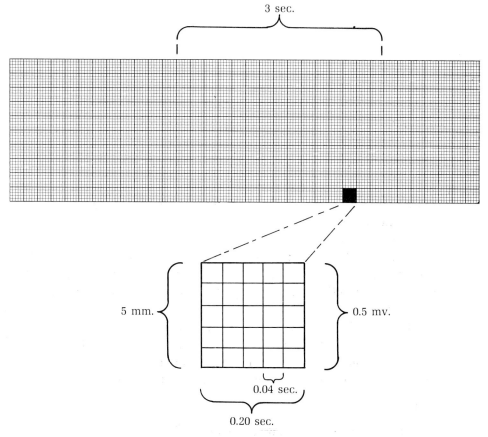

Fig. 5-10. ECG grid.

ECG PAPER

Time is measured on the horizontal plane. Each small square on the ECG paper represents 1 millimeter (mm.) in length and 0.04 second in time. The larger square that is defined by the heavier line represents 5 mm. in length and 0.2 second in time.

Amplitude (voltage) is measured on the vertical plane. All diagnostic twelve-lead ECGs are standardized so that 1 mv. is equal to 10 mm. (two large squares).

The single vertical lines above the ECG grid represent 3-inch or 3-second intervals (Fig. 5-10).

CALCULATION OF HEART RATE

ECG tracings may be used to calculate heart rate as follows:

1 Count the number of cycles in a 6-inch strip and multiply by 10. This method can be used when the rhythm is either regular or irregular.
2 Count the number of large squares between two R waves and divide into 300. This method is accurate only if the rhythm is regular.
3 Measure the time interval in seconds between two R waves and divide into 60. For example, if the distance between R waves of two consecutive beats if 0.60 second, the heart rate is 100. This method is accurate only if the rhythm is regular.
4 For more rapid rhythms or to calculate a rapid atrial rate, count the number of small squares (0.04 second) between R waves or P waves and divide into 1500. This method is accurate only if the rhythm is regular.

MEANING AND DURATION OF ECG INTERVALS

The *P-R interval* (Fig. 5-11) is normally between 0.12 and 0.2 second. It represents the length of time from the beginning of atrial activation to the beginning of ventricular activation. It is measured from the beginning of the P wave to the first ventricular deflection.

The *QRS duration* (Fig. 5-11) is normally between 0.06 and 0.10 second. It represents ventricular conduction time and is measured from the beginning of ventricular activity to its completion, when the graph returns again to the isoelectric line.

The *Q-T interval* (Fig. 5-11) varies with the heart rate and represents electrical systole. It is measured from the onset of ventricular activity to the end of the T wave. With average heart rates of between 60 and 80 per minute, the Q-T interval is normally not over 0.38 second.

ARTIFACTS

An artifact is any product on the ECG that is not due to the currents generated during the cardiac cycle. Artifacts include alternating current (AC)

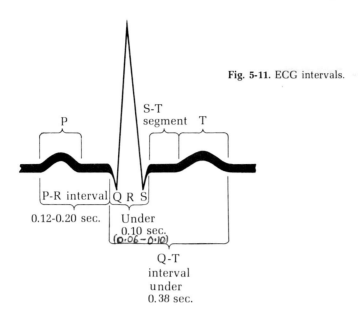

Fig. 5-11. ECG intervals.

interference, somatic tremor, wandering base line, standardization, and external cardiac massage.

AC interference

AC interference is caused by leakage of the electric power used in the hospital or office. This current pulses or alternates at exactly 60 cycles per second. A magnifying glass will show exactly sixty even, regular spikes in a 1-second interval (Fig. 5-12).

Somatic tremor

Body tremor presents an entirely different picture (Fig. 5-13). There is a grossly uneven, tremulous base line. It is often seen in patients experiencing tension—the electrical potentials of their "tensed" muscles are picked up by the electrodes.

Wandering base line

A wandering base line is an artifact in which the complexes are present but the base line is undulating (Fig. 5-14).

Standardization

An artifact deliberately introduced by the operator so that the interpreter can compare the relationship of the complexes with a known electrical stimulus (Fig. 5-15) is called a standardization artifact. A 1 mv. stimulus should cause the stylette to deflect 10 mm. (two large squares). If it does not, the operator adjusts the controls until this result is achieved.

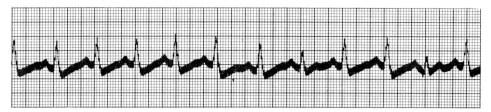

Fig. 5-12. AC interference.

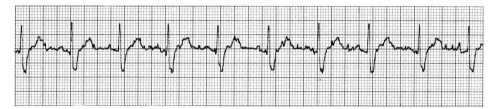

Fig. 5-13. Somatic tremor.

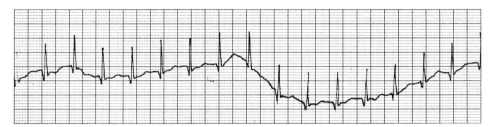

Fig. 5-14. Wandering base line.

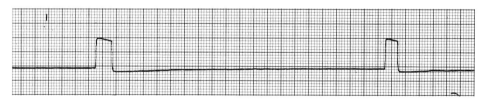

Fig. 5-15. Standardization.

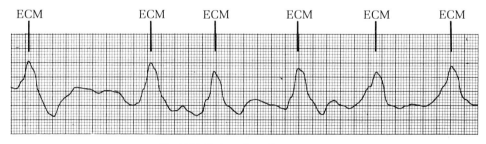

Fig. 5-16. External cardiac massage.

External cardiac massage

The complexes sometimes produced by external cardiac massage (ECM) may resemble regular, broad ventricular beats (Fig. 5-16).

SUMMARY

The normal ECG is composed of a P wave, a QRS complex, and a T wave. The morphology of these deflections is dependent upon the orientation of the cardiac vector to the lead axis. The deflections are recorded on grid paper that measures time and amplitude (voltage). The strength of the vector, its direction, and its speed are thus measured.

STUDY HELPS

1 Draw the normal wave deflections of the ECG.
2 Indicate the direction of the QRS deflections (positive or negative) for the Q wave, the R wave, and the S wave.
3 What determines the shape of the P wave and the QRS complex?
4 What is meant by the term "R wave progression"?
5 Explain the electrophysiology of the T wave.
6 Draw the normal ECG and indicate the absolute and relative refractory periods.
7 Why is the relative refractory period also called the vulnerable period?
8 ECG paper is designed to measure time and amplitude. Explain how this is done.
9 What is meant by "standardization"?
10 How would you calculate the heart rate in an irregular rhythm? A regular rhythm? A very rapid atrial rate?
11 What is represented by the P-R interval? The QRS interval? What are the normal values?
12 Define "artifact" and list those most commonly seen.

6 Arrhythmias originating in the sinus node

NORMAL ATRIAL DEPOLARIZATION

The thin-walled muscle of the atrium produces a weak vector. This is recorded on the ECG as a small P wave, which in some leads may be barely visible. Impulses originating in the sinus node will travel the same pathway through the atria each time. Therefore the atrial vector will normally be of uniform strength and direction, so that all of the P waves in one lead will be identical in shape (Fig. 6-1).

ARRHYTHMIAS ORIGINATING IN THE SINUS NODE

Normally the sinus node depolarizes at regular intervals, between 60 and 100 times per minute. If the rate of depolarization is irregular, too fast, too slow, or fails to produce a sufficiently strong stimulus, an arrhythmia is present (Fig. 6-2).

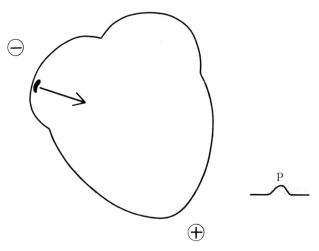

Fig. 6-1. P vector related to a monitoring lead axis and the resultant deflection.

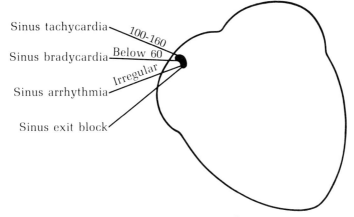

Fig. 6-2. Arrhythmias originating in the sinus node.

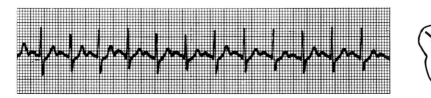

Fig. 6-3. Sinus tachycardia.

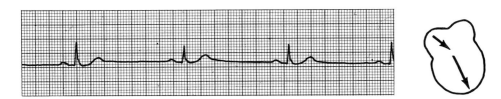

Fig. 6-4. Sinus bradycardia.

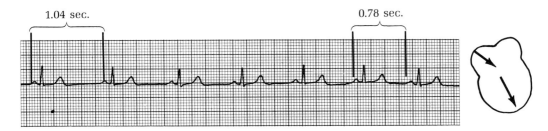

Fig. 6-5. Sinus arrhythmia.

Sinus tachycardia

In sinus tachycardia the impulses originate regularly as they should in the sinus node. The current travels along its usual path through the atria and ventricles. The rate, however, is faster than normal (100 to 160). The tracing in Fig. 6-3 shows a rate of 140 per minute. The pacemaker is the sinus node and conduction is normal.

Sinus bradycardia

In sinus bradycardia the pacemaker is the sinus node and conduction is normal. The rhythm is regular, but the rate, below 60, is too slow. In the tracing shown in Fig. 6-4 the rate is 38 per minute.

Sinus arrhythmia

The pacemaker is the sinus node and conduction is normal in sinus arrhythmia. However, the rhythm is irregular. Sinus arrhythmias are those conditions in which the difference between the shortest P-P interval and the longest P-P interval is greater than 0.12 second. These variations in rate are usually due to the vagal effect of respiration on the heart. The rate increases with inspiration and decreases with expiration.

The difference between the two intervals marked in Fig. 6-5 is 0.26 second. It is a sinus arrhythmia. The rate is normal at 75.

Sinus exit block

When a P wave fails to appear as it should, the terms "sinus arrest" and "sinoatrial block" have been used. The term "sinus arrest" implies that all of the pacemaker cells in the sinus node have failed momentarily. There are thousands of these specialized cells in the sinus node, and it is highly improbable that all of them would fail temporarily at the same time. The second term, "sinoatrial block," implies that the conduction pathway from the sinus node to the atrial musculature has been blocked. Apart from the special preferential pathways connecting the sinus node with the atrial musculature, there are many fibers that supplement these pathways. It is therefore improbable that impulse conduction would be blocked temporarily in all of the fibers at once.

The exact mechanism of sinus arrest or sinoatrial block is unknown. However, it is probable that the sinus node continues to depolarize but fails to generate an impulse that is strong enough to leave the sinus node. The term "exit block" is used to describe the condition in which other parts of the heart have areas with weak action potentials. "Sinus exit block," then, describes the mechanism thought to be responsible for a momentary failure of the sinus node to deliver its impulse to the atria.

Usually a single impulse fails to conduct to the atria (Fig. 6-6). Since the

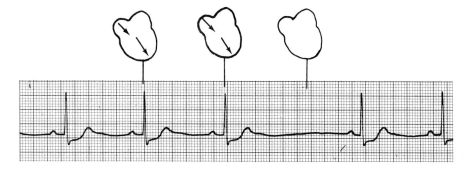

Fig. 6-6. Sinus exit block.

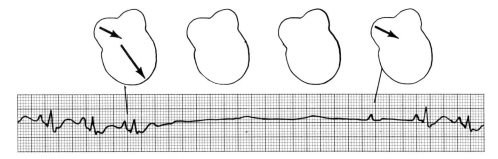

Fig. 6-7. Sinus exit block and atrial standstill.

basic rate is 52, this is also a sinus bradycardia. If the exit block continues for a longer time, atrial standstill results.

Fig. 6-7 illustrates the abrupt failure of conduction from the sinus node to the atrial musculature. The atria remain inactive for a little over 3½ seconds (atrial standstill). There is no activity in either the atria or the ventricles during this time. When conduction from the sinus node to the atrium is finally resumed, the ventricle does not respond immediately.

SUMMARY

The arrhythmias originating in the sinus node are sinus tachycardia, sinus bradycardia, sinus arrhythmia, and sinus exit block. In all of these arrhythmias the sinus node, as it should be, is the pacemaker of the heart. However, its rate is either too fast, too slow, irregular, or inconsistent.

TEST TRACINGS

Figs. 6-8 to 6-11 are the ECG test tracings of arrhythmias that we have just studied. In this exercise, ascertain the following facts:

    1 What is the rate?

    2 Is the rhythm regular?

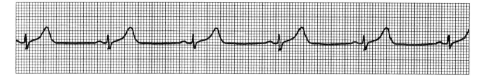

Fig. 6-8

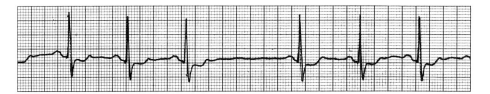

Fig. 6-9

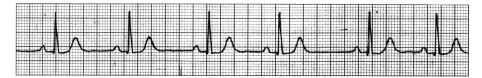

Fig. 6-10

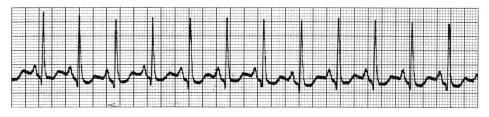

Fig. 6-11

Notice the difference between the irregularity caused by a sinus arrhythmia and the irregularity characteristic of a sinus arrest.

ANSWERS

6-8 *Sinus bradycardia.* The rate is 48. Rhythm is regular and conduction is normal.

6-9 *Sinus exit block.* The sinus node has depolarized but has failed to conduct this impulse to the atria. This failure results in the absence of a P wave.

6-10 *Sinus arrhythmia.* The rhythm is irregular. The P-P interval at the beginning of the tracing is a full large square (0.20 second), shorter than the P-P interval at the end of the tracing. The rate is approximately 60 per minute. Conduction is normal.

6-11 *Sinus tachycardia.* The rate of the sinus node is 110. Conduction is normal.

7 Atrial ectopics

TERMINOLOGY

ectopic beat   Arises from a focus outside the sinus node.

extrasystole   Has its origin outside the sinus node; premature beat is usually termed an extra-systole; ectopic beat is not necessarily premature.

active rhythms   Begin prematurely, assuming control even when the normal pacemaker is adequate.

passive rhythms   Not premature; appear usually when the normal mechanism fails or slows excessively.

bigeminal rhythms   Occur in two's; term is used when an ectopic beat is coupled to the preceding sinus beat and the pattern is repeated through the strip.

trigeminal rhythms   Occur in three's; may be either two normal beats coupled with an ectopic beat or two ectopic beats coupled with a normal complex; pattern is repeated through the strip.

INTRODUCTION

When an ectopic focus is active in either atrium, it can cause a number of arrhythmias, depending upon its irritability (Fig. 7-1). Occasionally the premature atrial contraction may take over as pacemaker with a series of stimuli that begins and ends abruptly, called paroxysmal atrial tachycardia. Atrial tachycardia is the term given to such a series of stimuli if it is sustained. A more irritable ectopic focus causes atrial stimulation at a more rapid rate. This may cause atrial flutter. If the rate of this stimulus exceeds 350 or 400 per minute, the atria will be unable to respond with organized electrical activity, and the resultant disorganized activity is known as atrial fibrillation.

P′ WAVE

When the atrial impulse originates at a point other than the sinus node, the resultant deflection is called a P′ (P prime) wave. The ectopic focus may be anywhere in the atria. The shape of the P′ wave will depend upon the orientation of the vector to the axis of the lead (Fig. 7-2). If the ectopic focus is in the vicinity of the sinus node, the resultant P′ wave will closely resemble the normal sinus P wave. Its sole distinguishing feature may be that it is premature. However, if the ectopic focus is located so that its vector takes a different path, the resultant P′ wave will have a different shape than the normal sinus P wave.

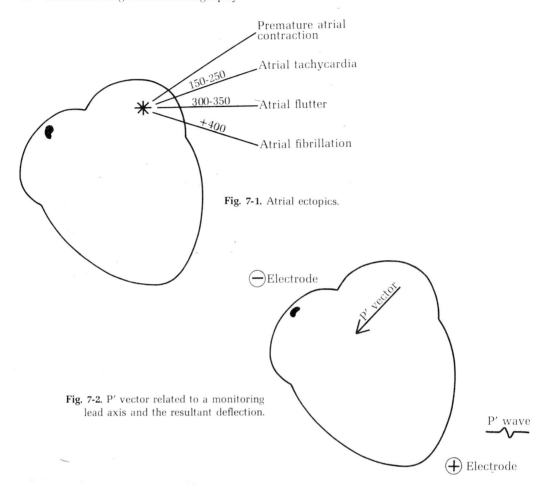

Fig. 7-1. Atrial ectopics.

Fig. 7-2. P′ vector related to a monitoring
lead axis and the resultant deflection.

PREMATURE ATRIAL CONTRACTION (PAC)

If an ectopic focus in the atria is to usurp control from a normally functioning sinus node, it must do so prematurely, before the atrial tissue becomes depolarized by the normal sinus stimulus. Such a usurpation results
in a PAC.

Fig. 7-3 depicts sinus bradycardia with a rate of 48. Mark off the first
two normal sinus P waves. Bring this mark across the strip, and you will
easily find the premature atrial complex. It occurs early, before the expected
sinus P wave. It is also shaped differently, being a little narrower and more
pointed than the normal sinus P waves. Because of the slow rate of the sinus
node, this ectopic focus has a greater opportunity to intrude into the normal rhythm.

The PACs in Fig. 7-4 are hidden in the preceding T waves. Ectopic P
waves (P′) commonly hide in T waves. Whenever there is an irregularity, it

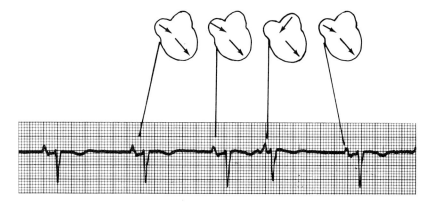

Fig. 7-3. Single premature atrial contraction (PAC).

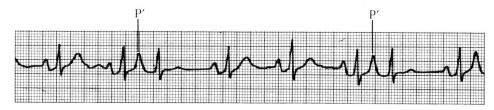

Fig. 7-4. PAC hidden in the T wave.

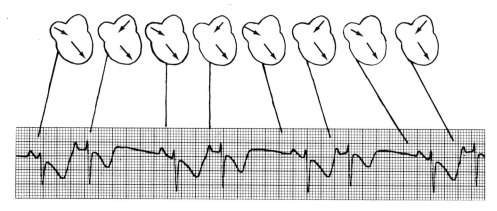

Fig. 7-5. Bigeminal PACs.

is well to closely examine and compare the T waves. They should all be the same shape. In Fig. 7-4 there are two T waves that are more pointed and peaked than the others. They have been distorted by P′ waves and are followed by a normal ventricular response.

Bigeminal PACs

In Fig. 7-5 every other P wave is ectopic. Each P′ wave is followed by a normal ventricular response.

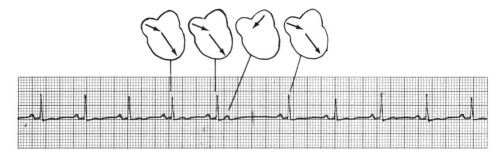

Fig. 7-6. Nonconducted PAC.

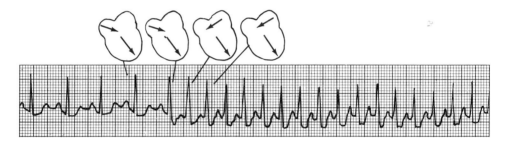

Fig. 7-7. Atrial tachycardia.

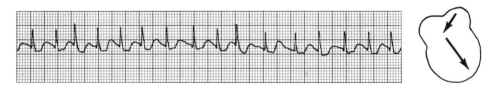

Fig. 7-8. Supraventricular tachycardia.

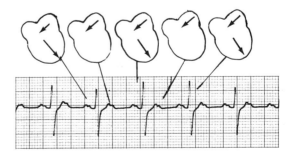

Fig. 7-9. Atrial tachycardia with 2:1 A-V conduction.

Nonconducted PACs

Again mark off the first two normal sinus P waves shown in Fig. 7-6 on a separate piece of paper. Bring this mark across the strip. At the point at which the rhythm becomes irregular, a P′ wave can be seen on the T wave. You may think this is only a T wave until you carefully examine and compare it with the T waves following the other complexes. They are flatter and not as pointed. The ventricular response to this ectopic P wave is absent. Conduction is blocked because of a physiological refractoriness in the ventricles. The PAC occurs before the ventricles are ready to accept it. Therefore this atrial stimulus is not conducted.

ATRIAL TACHYCARDIA

In atrial tachycardia a pacemaker in the atria governs the heart at a rate of 150 to 250 per minute.

Since the onset of this arrhythmia in Fig. 7-7 is visible, a diagnosis of atrial tachycardia is easily made. The tachycardia begins with a PAC. This ectopic focus then assumes control of the heart.

Mark off two normal sinus P waves on a piece of paper. In bringing these marks across the tracing and "walking out" the P waves, you will clearly see the P′ wave at the onset of the tachycardia. The sinus rate is 118 (sinus tachycardia). The rate of the atrial ectopic focus is approximately 222.

In Fig. 7-8 it is difficult to tell if the ectopic focus is in the atria or in the A-V junction since P waves are not seen. However, it is certain that it is supraventricular, or above the bifurcation of the bundle of His, since the ventricular complexes are of normal duration. The arrhythmia is therefore called a *supraventricular tachycardia*.

Atrial tachycardia with block

Normal hearts are able to respond to atrial rates that are as rapid as 200 per minute with 1:1 A-V conduction. There will usually be a functional A-V block when the atrial rate exceeds this limit.

In Fig. 7-9 two P′ waves can be seen between each QRS complex. Mark off two consecutive P′ waves. Bring this interval along the tracing and you will find that the P′ waves occur at regular intervals. The atrial rate is 184. The ventricular rate is 92.

Paroxysmal atrial tachycardia (PAT)

When an atrial ectopic focus dominates the heart in bursts of five or more, it is termed a PAT. When the paroxysm terminates, the sinus node once again regains control.

In Fig. 7-10 a single PAC interrupts the sinus rhythm. A series of PACs then occurs, after which the sinus node paces the heart. This burst of tachycardia is called PAT.

ATRIAL FLUTTER

This arrhythmia, like atrial tachycardia, is caused by an irritable focus somewhere in the atria. The atria are stimulated even more rapidly, at a rate somewhere between 300 and 350. The atria have been known to respond in a unified fashion even to a rate of 400 or more.

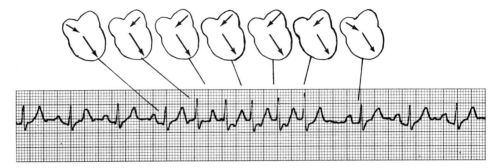

Fig. 7-10. Paroxysmal atrial tachycardia.

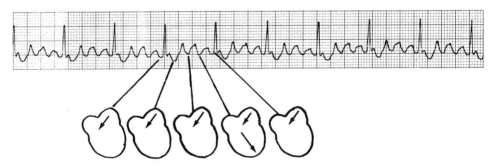

Fig. 7-11. Atrial flutter with 4:1 A-V conduction.

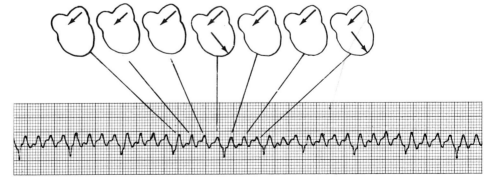

Fig. 7-12. Atrial flutter with variable block.

Atrial flutter defined—rate versus shape

There are some who, claiming that there is no distinction at all between atrial tachycardia and atrial flutter, call both a supraventricular tachycardia. They maintain that the quicker the atrial discharge, the more likely the P′ waves will assume the typical sawtooth pattern of atrial flutter.

Others claim that the distinction between atrial tachycardia and atrial flutter lies solely in the shape of the complexes. They say that the characteristic undulating sawtooth pattern is atrial flutter regardless of rate and that when there is an isoelectric line between P′ waves, the arrhythmia is atrial tachycardia.

For our purposes the rate and morphology will determine the name given to the arrhythmia, so that rates of 150 to 250 will be termed *atrial tachycardia,* and rates of 300 to 350 or more will be termed *atrial flutter.* The "gray area" in between 250 and 300 will be classified according to morphology.

Atrial flutter with "block"

Here the term "block" is used to indicate a "functional" rather than a pathological block. The ventricles are protected from rapid atrial rates by the refractory state of the A-V junction.

The tracing in Fig. 7-11 is an example of atrial flutter with 4:1 A-V conduction (block). The atrial rate is 325 per minute and the characteristic undulating, sawtooth pattern may be observed. There is a response to every fourth P′ wave; thus the ventricular rate is 80.

Atrial flutter with variable block

In Fig. 7-12 the ventricles are irregular in their response to a rapid (350 per minute) atrial stimulus. Responses of 2:1, 3:1, and 4:1 can be seen in this tracing.

Atrial flutter with a high degree of block

When the block at the A-V node exceeds 4:1, there may be a pathological cause rather than a functional refractoriness.

In Fig. 7-13 the atrial rate is 300, and the ventricles are beating regularly at a rate of 55. There is no constant relationship between the QRS and the preceding flutter wave, indicating that the ventricle is beating independently.

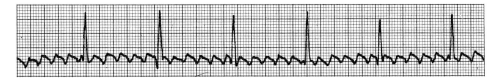

Fig. 7-13. Atrial flutter with a high degree of block.

Morphology of the flutter wave

In atrial flutter the atrial repolarization wave (Ta wave) is clearly seen. In the normal sinus rhythm it is hidden in the QRS complex.

The P′ wave is usually the negative deflection of the sawtooth pattern. The Ta wave (atrial repolarization) is the positive deflection (Fig. 7-14).

In atrial flutter the atria beat rapidly and regularly. Therefore a QRS complex may occur at the same time as a P′ (flutter) wave. In order to determine the degree of block, it is important to mark off the two or three visible P′ waves. In bringing these marks along the tracing, you will find a P′ wave hidden within the QRS complex.

ATRIAL FIBRILLATION

The atria can respond in an organized fashion to as many as 350 and sometimes as many as 400 or more impulses per minute. With a more rapid stimulus, the atrial muscle cells cannot all repolarize in time for the next stimulus. As a result, the ectopic vector is rejected by the refractory cells, and electrical chaos results. Depolarization and repolarization will occur, but there will be no unified electrical activity. Rather there are vectors in different directions at different times (Fig. 7-15).

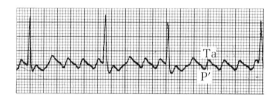

Fig. 7-14. Morphology of P′ wave in atrial flutter.

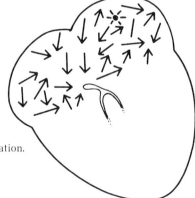

Fig. 7-15. Disorganized electrical activity of atrial fibrillation.

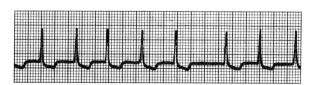

Fig. 7-16. Atrial fibrillation with a fine isoelectric line.

Fibrillatory line

At times the ECG electrodes will sense none of these disorganized, rampant vectors. The isoelectric line will then appear almost flat and is referred to as "fine fibrillation" (Fig. 7-16).

At other times the ECG electrodes will sense some of this vagrant electrical activity, which will be recorded as a coarse fibrillatory line ("coarse fibrillation"), indicative only of disorganized electrical activity (Fig. 7-17).

When the fibrillatory line is coarse, as in Fig. 7-17, you may at times see what you think might be a P wave. Keep in mind the fact that true P waves are regular, all of the same configuration, and usually occurring at the same place before each QRS complex.

Atrial fibrillation and A-V conduction

Thus far we have established that in atrial fibrillation the P waves are absent. There is either a completely flat isoelectric line or disorganized electrical activity in the form of a wavy fibrillatory line with no set pattern.

Normally the A-V node is depolarized regularly by an impulse arriving from the sinus node. In atrial fibrillation there are many vectors (depolarization waves or currents) bombarding the A-V node. Some of the action potentials stimulating the A-V node are weak. They are therefore not propagated into the ventricles, although they do partially depolarize the A-V junction, leaving it refractory to another stimulus (concealed conduction). Thus the ventricular response in atrial fibrillation is irregular and as rapid as A-V junctional recovery will allow.

The ventricular response shown in the tracing of atrial fibrillation in Fig. 7-18 is approximately 140 per minute.

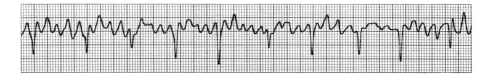

Fig. 7-17. Atrial fibrillation with a coarse fibrillatory line.

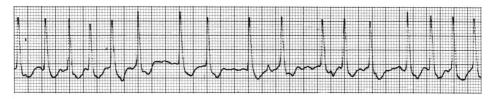

Fig. 7-18. Atrial fibrillation with an uncontrolled ventricular response.

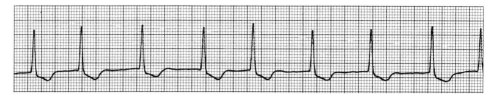

Fig. 7-19. Atrial fibrillation with a controlled ventricular response (digitalis effect).

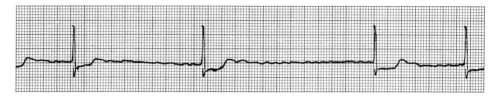

Fig. 7-20. Atrial fibrillation with a slow ventricular response.

Fig. 7-19 illustrates a controlled atrial fibrillation. The ventricular response has been slowed to 90 by the action of digitalis on the A-V node.

Fig. 7-20 is an example of atrial fibrillation with a slow ventricular response of 40. A fine fibrillatory line is visible between the R waves.

CORONARY SINUS AS AN ECTOPIC FOCUS

The coronary sinus lies in the coronary sulcus and is about 1½ inches long. It opens into the right atrium just next to the orifice of the inferior vena cava (Fig. 7-21). Most of the coronary venous blood from the left ventricle empties into it.

Because of its close proximity to the A-V node, an ectopic focus at the orifice of the coronary sinus would cause a nodal-type P′ wave (inverted in leads II, III, and aV$_F$). The P′-R interval would, however, be 0.12 second or more.

The negative P′ wave in Fig. 7-22 indicates that the vector is directed upward, away from the positive terminal of lead II. The P′-R interval is abnormally long (0.24 second), indicating that the impulse must have met with the normal conduction delay at the A-V node. Therefore the focus must be above this point. Because of the enhanced automaticity in the area of the coronary sinus, the ectopic focus is thought to be located here rather than on the floor of the right atrium. However, it is also possible that the impulse originated from the cells surrounding the A-V node.

WANDERING PACEMAKER

The wandering pacemaker is a passive rather than an active arrhythmia and refers to the atrial escape as opposed to the PAC. A shifting or wander-

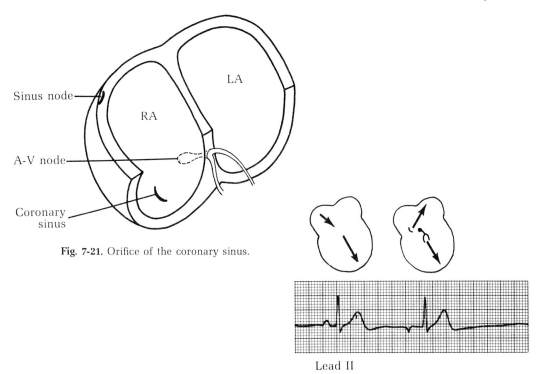

Fig. 7-21. Orifice of the coronary sinus.

Lead II

Fig. 7-22. PAC (coronary sinus).

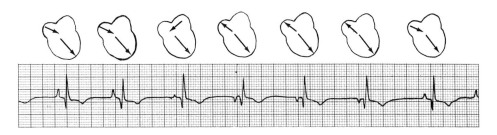

Fig. 7-23. Wandering pacemaker.

ing pacemaker is characterized by a P-P' interval that is longer than the normal P-P interval.

In Fig. 7-23 the pacemaker shift is easily seen as the P wave deflection changes from positive to negative. The P-P' interval is 0.09 second longer than the P-P interval. The ectopic pacemaker is therefore not active and premature (PAC) but late and passive. The first P' wave is biphasic, indicating either a third ectopic pacemaker somewhere between the sinus and A-V nodes or an atrial fusion beat (a collision of sinus and nodal vectors).

Pacemaker shifts may be caused by almost identical intrinsic rates in both nodes. Thus if the sinus node slows down, the A-V junction or another focus may depolarize first.

SUMMARY

In this chapter you have learned that the P wave can be generated at a point other than the sinus node. When the atria are depolarized from an ectopic focus, one of a number of arrhythmias may result, depending upon the degree of irritability and the location of the ectopic focus.

All atrial ectopics are diagnosed by observing P waves or noting their absence. The P′ wave generated by an active ectopic focus (PAC) is early and usually of a different shape from the sinus P wave. The P′ wave generated by a passive ectopic focus (wandering pacemaker) is not premature. An atrial ectopic focus taking over at a rate of 150 to 250 is called atrial tachycardia. If the rate is 300 to 350 or more, the condition is atrial flutter and usually has a characteristic sawtooth pattern. When the stimuli occur so rapidly that the atria cannot respond in an organized fashion, the result is atrial fibrillation. This condition is characterized by the absence of P waves and irregular ventricular response.

If there is an ectopic focus in the coronary sinus, the P′ wave will be negative in leads II, III, and aV_F, and the P′-R interval will be 0.12 second or more.

TEST TRACINGS

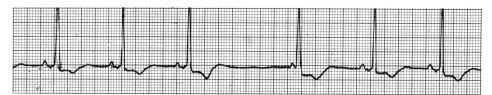

Fig. 7-24

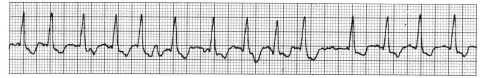

Fig. 7-25

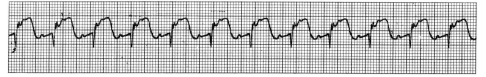

Fig. 7-26

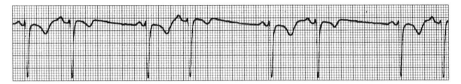

Fig. 7-27

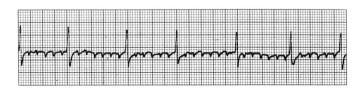

Fig. 7-28

ANSWERS

7-24 *Sinus exit block with junctional escape.* This regular sinus rhythm is interrupted by a pause when an anticipated P wave does not occur (sinus exit block). The first P wave after the pause does not conduct to the ventricles because the P-R interval is too short for conduction. There is a junctional escape beat. Since the A-V junction was not activated by the sinus node, self-excitation occurred.

7-25 *Atrial fibrillation.* Here again the absence of P waves and an irregular ventricular response make a diagnosis of atrial fibrillation certain.

7-26 *Atrial tachycardia with 2:1 A-V conduction.* The atrial rate is 200. There are two P′ waves for every QRS complex, yielding a ventricular rate of 100. One P′ wave is apparent just before the QRS complex. The other is on the S-T segment.

7-27 *Bigeminal PACs.* Every other P wave is premature.

7-28 *Atrial flutter.* The characteristic sawtooth pattern of atrial flutter is immediately apparent in this tracing. There is a high degree of block that may be due to the unusually rapid atrial rate (428) rather than to a pathological block.

8 Ventricular ectopics

ACTIVE VENTRICULAR EXTRASYSTOLES

Myocardial ischemia or infarction, fear, emotional tension, and a variety of factors can all cause irritable foci in the ventricles to depolarize prematurely (before the expected stimulus from the sinus node). This is an *active* mechanism usurping control and a function of phase 4 of the action potential.

PASSIVE ESCAPE BEATS

An alteration of the rhythm or conduction ability of the special conductive system of the heart, such as a slowing of the sinus node or an occluding lesion of the A-V junction, may force an ectopic pacemaker to assume control of the ventricle. The ectopic pacemaker assumes control only because of the failure of the normal pacemaker and not because of its own excitability. This is therefore a *passive* escape mechanism.

NORMAL VENTRICULAR DEPOLARIZATION

Since V_1 and V_6 are on opposite sides of the heart, a current that is reflected as a positive event in V_1 will be inscribed as a negative event in V_6. For example, the major ventricular vector is normally directed to the left, toward V_6. This event will therefore be reflected as a positive deflection in V_6 and as a negative deflection in V_1.

The sequence of depolarization of the ventricles (Fig. 8-1) is as follows:

Event No. 1. After it traverses the A-V junction, the impulse depolarizes the interventricular (I-V) septum. A small current moves from left to right, causing a flow toward the V_1 electrode. An r wave is written. The current flows away from the V_6 electrode, causing a small q wave to be written.

Event No. 2. The ventricular muscle mass is the next to depolarize. Because the left ventricle is larger, the main electrical force will be leftward and inferior. This is a movement away from the V_1 electrode; thus an S wave is written. The current flow is toward the V_6 electrode, and an R wave is written.

Event No. 3. The epicardial surface at the base of the heart is the last

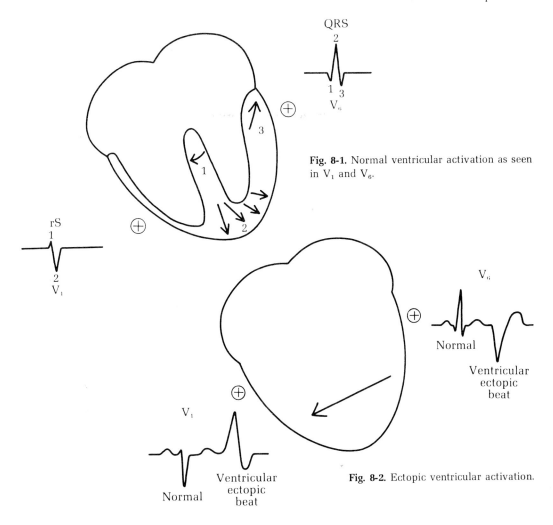

Fig. 8-1. Normal ventricular activation as seen in V_1 and V_6.

Fig. 8-2. Ectopic ventricular activation.

to depolarize, the sequence being as follows: the pulmonary conus, posterobasal portion of the left ventricle, and uppermost epicardial portion of the I-V septum. This may or may not be recorded in V_1 as a small r wave. In V_6 this small vector flowing away from the electrode is recorded as an s wave.

DEPOLARIZATION FOLLOWING A VENTRICULAR ECTOPIC STIMULUS

An ectopic focus stimulating the ventricles will almost always be located within the His-Purkinje system. The ventricular vector will begin at the site of the focus and travel toward the rest of the ventricular muscle mass. The orientation of this vector to the axes of the leads will be abnormal, causing an abnormal and different deflection. Because the impulse cannot travel on its usual accelerated path via the bundle of His and bundle branches, conduction will be delayed, causing a characteristically broad complex.

The shape of a ventricular extrasystole is dependent upon the location of the ectopic focus in the ventricles and upon the orientation of the vector to the axis of the lead (Fig. 8-2).

OTHER CHARACTERISTICS OF THE VENTRICULAR EXTRASYSTOLE

Apart from its being broad and distorted, there are other means of recognizing the premature ventricular contraction (PVC): prematurity, full compensatory pause, increased amplitude, T wave of opposite polarity, and no related P wave.

Prematurity

An ectopic focus must depolarize the ventricle before the normal sinus stimulus arrives. The active ventricular extrasystole is therefore always premature.

Full compensatory pause

When a PVC occurs, the atrium is usually not affected. The sinus node continues to beat regularly. The P waves will therefore occur on time in spite of the ventricular irregularity. There will be no ventricular response to the P wave approximate to the PVC because the ventricle will be in a refractory period and thus unable to respond. There will, however, be a response to the following P wave. This sequence causes what is called a full compensatory pause.

Notice that the P waves in Fig. 8-3 fall right on time in spite of the interruption of the normal ventricular rhythm by the PVC.

To measure a full compensatory pause, mark off three normal cycles. Then place the first mark on the P wave of the normal cycle preceding the PVC. The third mark should fall exactly on the P wave following the ventricular ectopic beat.

Increased amplitude

The greater amplitude usually demonstrated by the PVC is caused by a stronger vector, the result of a greater number of depolarized (negative) cells opposing polarized (positive) cells.

The normal cardiac vector passes along the anatomical axis of the heart, which is diagrammatically illustrated in Fig. 8-4.

The usual sequence of electrical events in the heart causes an equalization of the electrical charges. The endocardium depolarizes before the epicardium. Thus there are fewer negative and positive charges opposing each other than there would be if the whole top half of the heart depolarized before the lower half.

The vector from an ectopic focus often has a deviated axis traveling across the width of the heart (Fig. 8-5). One side of the heart, at the location

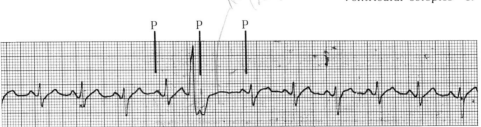

No QRS
(refactory)

P   P   P

Fig. 8-3. Full compensatory pause.

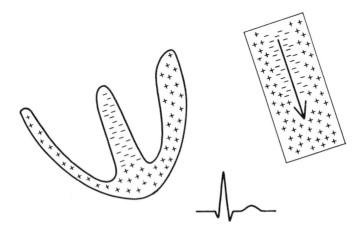

Fig. 8-4. Normal depolarization.

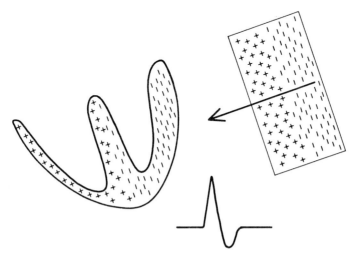

Fig. 8-5. Abnormal depolarization.

of the ectopic focus, depolarizes before the other. This results in a greater number of negative cells in the presence of positive cells. The resultant stronger vector is reflected in the ECG tracing by a complex of higher amplitude than the complex of the dominant sinus rhythm.

This strong vector of the PVC does not mean that the premature muscle contraction is stronger than normal. On the contrary, it will be weaker because it occurs early and has not allowed for complete ventricular filling and because the contraction following this errant stimulus will not be uniform.

Because of the compensatory pause following the PVC, there will be greater ventricular filling. Therefore the first normal beat following the PVC will be more forceful.

T wave of opposite polarity

Normally repolarization occurs from epicardium to endocardium, beginning at the apex of the heart—just the opposite to the normal depolarization process (Fig. 8-6).

Since current flows from negative to positive, a normal repolarization process will result in an upright T wave.

Conversely, the abnormal repolarization process will follow the same sequence as did the abnormal depolarization process because during delayed or abnormal depolarization, the cells at the apex are not activated soon enough to enable them to begin to repolarize first. Therefore the first cells to depolarize will be the first cells to repolarize (Fig. 8-7).

Since the direction of the two processes (depolarization and repolarization) is the same, the polarity of the two deflections will be opposite (the T wave will be of opposite polarity).

No related P wave

The ventricular ectopic contraction will not be associated with atrial activity. Thus, although a P wave may immediately precede a PVC, it will not be the cause of the ectopic ventricular activity.

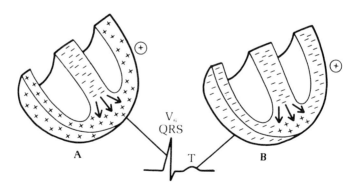

Fig. 8-6. A, Normal depolarization. **B,** Normal repolarization.

TYPES OF PREMATURE VENTRICULAR CONTRACTIONS (PVCs)
End-diastolic PVC

If a ventricular ectopic beat occurs late in diastole, there will be a P wave immediately preceding but unrelated to it. This P-R interval will be shorter than the dominant P-R interval, and the ectopic complex will be premature. This type of PVC is termed end diastolic (Fig. 8-8).

Because there is a normal P wave immediately preceding the end-diastolic PVC, it is frequently misdiagnosed as a PAC with aberrant ventricular conduction, but the ventricular complex, not the P wave, is premature.

Unifocal PVCs

Since the PVCs shown in Fig. 8-9 are identical in form, it is evident that they originate from a single focus in the ventricle.

Ventricular bigeminy

Every other beat in the tracing shown in Fig. 8-10 is a PVC from the same focus. Each is coupled to the preceding normal complex.

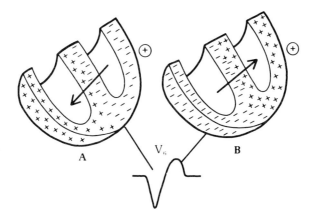

Fig. 8-7. A, Abnormal depolarization. **B,** Abnormal repolarization.

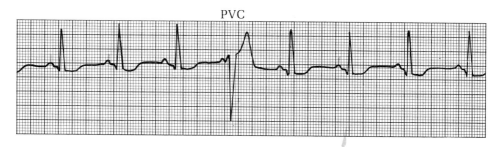

Fig. 8-8. End-diastolic premature ventricular contraction (PVC).

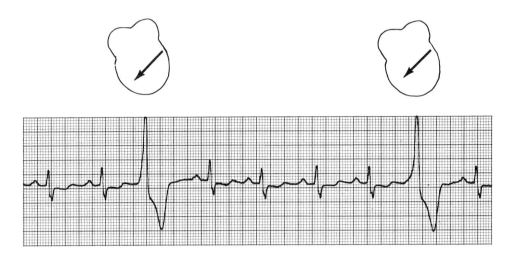

Fig. 8-9. Unifocal PVCs.

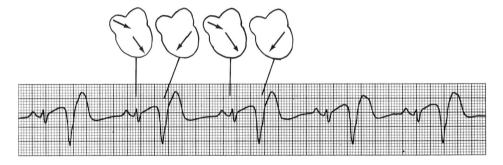

Fig. 8-10. Ventricular bigeminy.

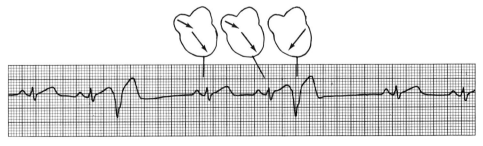

Fig. 8-11. Ventricular trigeminy.

Ventricular trigeminy

Ventricular trigeminy is a PVC characterized by rhythms that occur in groups of three. There may be one PVC for every two normal beats (Fig. 8-11) or two PVCs for each normal beat (Fig. 8-12).

Ventricular quadrigeminy

Fig. 8-13 is a tracing in which there are two ventricular ectopic beats for every two sinus-conducted complexes. When this pattern is repeated in any combination of four complexes, of which at least one is a ventricular ectopic beat, it is referred to as ventricular quadrigeminy.

PVCs WITH MORE SERIOUS IMPLICATIONS

Ventricular ectopic beats occurring in a diseased heart constitute a serious condition. There are, however, degrees of seriousness. Frequent, multifocal,

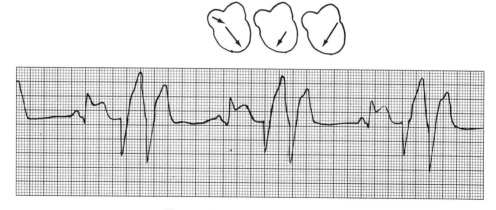

Fig. 8-12. Ventricular trigeminy.

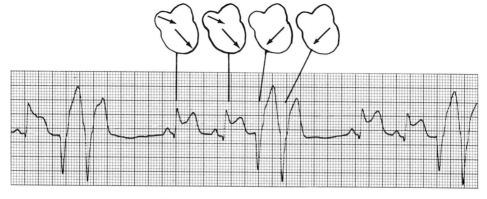

Fig. 8-13. Ventricular quadrigeminy.

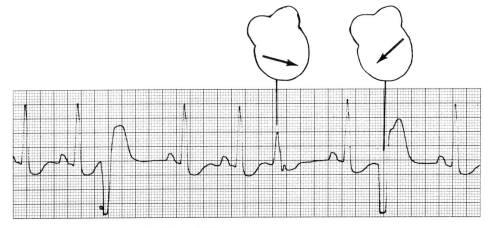

Fig. 8-14. Multifocal PVCs.

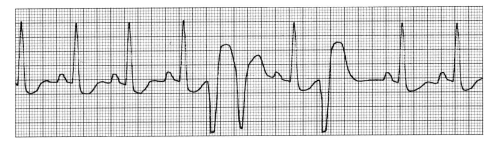

Fig. 8-15. Paired PVCs.

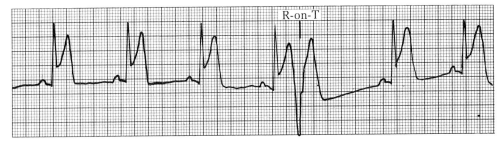

Fig. 8-16. R-on-T phenomenon.

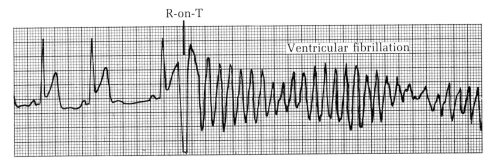

Fig. 8-17. R-on-T phenomenon causing ventricular fibrillation.

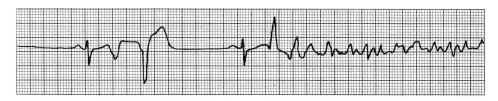

Fig. 8-18. Paired multifocal PVCs resulting in ventricular fibrillation.

left ventricular, and/or paired PVCs are more ominous than the occasional unifocal ventricular extrasystole. A PVC occurring during the relative refractory or vulnerable period would be even more ominous.

Multifocal PVCs

In the tracing shown in Fig. 8-14 there are two distinct contours to the PVCs, indicating that in each case the vector is oriented differently to the axis of the lead. There is more than one ectopic focus in the ventricles.

Paired PVCs

The PVCs in Fig. 8-15 occur in pairs, or "back to back." There is a very real danger that the second of the pair will meet with refractory tissue and result in electrical chaos.

R-on-T phenomenon

The term "R-on-T phenomenon" is used to indicate that an R wave (PVC) has occurred during the relative refractory period (on the T wave). Because the heart is not yet ready to respond to this stimulus in an organized fashion, a serious ventricular arrhythmia may result.

In Fig. 8-16 a PVC has occurred during the vulnerable period (on the T wave).

Again, in the same patient, Fig. 8-17 illustrates a PVC that falls on the T wave. The premature vector has stimulated a partially repolarized ventricle and has met with both nonrefractory and refractory tissue, resulting in electrical chaos, or ventricular fibrillation.

Fig. 8-18 shows a marked sinus bradycardia with coupled multifocal PVCs occurring on the T wave and resulting finally in ventricular fibrillation.

Left ventricular PVC

Ventricular ectopic beats that arise in the left ventricle are more serious than those arising in the right ventricle. The origin of the ectopic beat can be determined by the direction of the complex in V_1.

An ectopic vector proceeding from a focus in the left ventricle would travel toward the positive electrode of V_1, causing a positive deflection (right bundle branch block pattern) (Fig. 8-19).

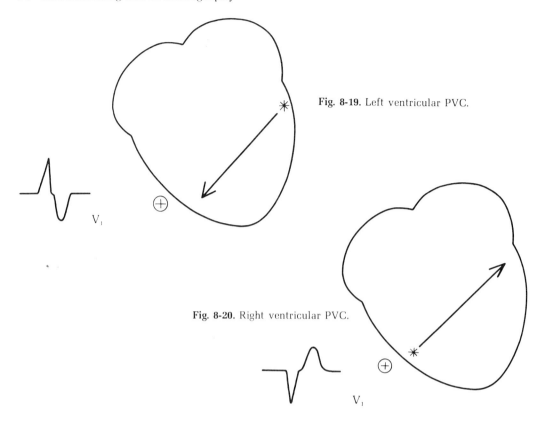

Fig. 8-19. Left ventricular PVC.

Fig. 8-20. Right ventricular PVC.

An ectopic vector proceeding from a focus in the right ventricle would travel away from the positive electrode of V_1, causing a negative deflection (left bundle branch block pattern) (Fig. 8-20).

EXCEPTIONS TO THE RULES

Ventricular extrasystoles are generally most easily recognized because of their full compensatory pause and the broadened complex that is so different in appearance from the normal sinus-conducted complexes. There are, however, exceptions to these rules. Two types of ventricular extrasystoles are not followed by the full compensatory pause. They are the interpolated extrasystole and the extrasystole with retrograde conduction to the atria. There are also two types that have a normal or almost normal appearance. They are the main-stem ectopic beat and the septal ectopic beat.

Interpolated extrasystole

This PVC is interposed (interpolated) between two normal sinus beats without disturbing the basic rhythm. The sinus node discharges normally, and the expected ventricular response is undisturbed. The interpolated extrasystole occurs only when the basic rate is so slow that it is physiologically

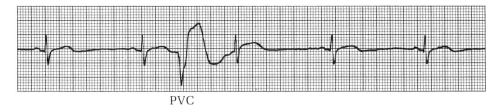

PVC

Fig. 8-21. Interpolated PVC.

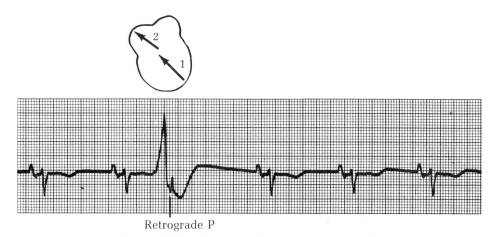

Retrograde P

Fig. 8-22. PVC with retrograde conduction to the atria.

possible to find the myocardium nonrefractory long enough to complete the response to an ectopic stimulus and return to the nonrefractory state before the next expected normal ventricular response.

The basic rate in the tracing shown in Fig. 8-21 is 47. In response to an ectopic stimulus, the ventricles are able to depolarize, repolarize, and return to a nonrefractory state before the next expected normal beat. Since the ventricular rhythm is uninterrupted, the interpolated PVC does not have a full compensatory pause.

Ventricular extrasystole with retrograde conduction

In most cases the depolarization current from the ectopic focus in the ventricle does not travel up the A-V junction to activate the atrium (retrograde conduction). When it does, the sinus node is depolarized early, and the next normal sinus stimulus will occur a little earlier than normal. This sequence of events will produce a less than full compensatory pause.

Fig. 8-22 is a tracing in which a negative P′ wave can be seen immediately following the PVC. In leads II, III, and aV$_F$, retrograde activation of the atria will cause a negative P′ wave. The pause following the PVC is not fully compensatory.

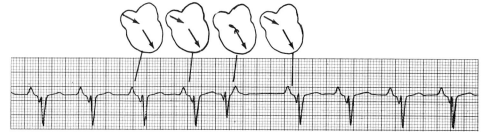

Fig. 8-23. Main-stem PVC.

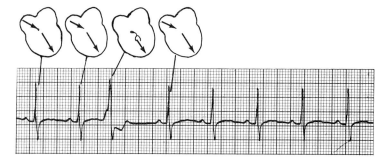

Fig. 8-24. Septal PVC.

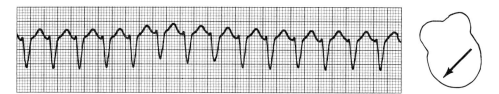

Fig. 8-25. Ventricular tachycardia.

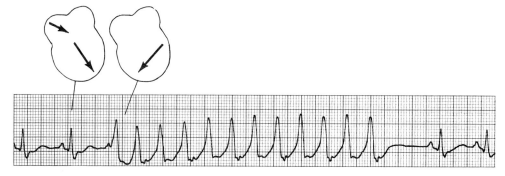

Fig. 8-26. Paroxysmal ventricular tachycardia.

Main-stem extrasystole

If the ectopic focus is in the main stem of the bundle of His, the resultant ventricular complex, though premature and ectopic, will appear normal in contour. Since the sinus node remains undisturbed, there will be a full compensatory pause. The location of this ectopic focus is the same as that of the junctional rhythms, but retrograde conduction to the atrium is blocked.

The ventricular extrasystole shown in Fig. 8-23 produces a contour that is identical to the contours of normal sinus-conducted beats. However, it is premature and is followed by a full compensatory pause, indicating that the ectopic focus is in the bundle of His and that retrograde conduction to the atria is blocked.

Septal extrasystole

This PVC arises from a focus in the I-V septum close to the point at which the bundle of His bifurcates (below the bifurcation). It is therefore called "septal."

The PVC shown in Fig. 8-24 has only a slightly different morphology from the sinus-conducted beats. It is followed by a full compensatory pause, indicating that the normal sinus rate has been undisturbed. This fact, coupled with its prematurity, classifies it as a PVC. The fact that its morphology is close to normal indicates that the ectopic focus is below the bifurcation of the bundle of His within the I-V septum.

VENTRICULAR TACHYCARDIA

Ventricular tachycardia is an arrhythmia characterized by an ectopic focus that dominates the ventricles. The ECG shows a continuous series of broad, rapid ventricular ectopic beats (Fig. 8-25).

PAROXYSMAL VENTRICULAR TACHYCARDIA

Paroxysmal ventricular tachycardia is a burst of tachycardia initiated by a PVC. In Fig. 8-26, eleven PVCs follow the initial premature beat, after which the tachycardia is terminated, and the sinus node is once again in command. Paroxysmal ventricular tachycardia, then, is a series of PVCs that ends spontaneously.

VENTRICULAR FIBRILLATION

Ventricular fibrillation involves electrical activity that is not unified. Individual muscle fibers are depolarizing, but they are disorganized and fail to produce a proper ventricular contraction. The heart quivers and twitches (Fig. 8-27).

The electrodes will record this erratic activity, as shown in Fig. 8-28. Coarse ventricular fibrillation (Fig. 8-28, *A*) indicates more electrical activity

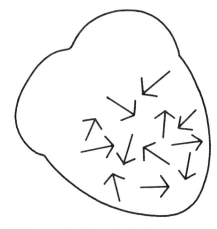

Fig. 8-27. Disorganized electrical activity of ventricular fibrillation.

A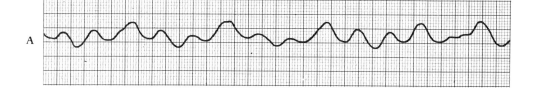

B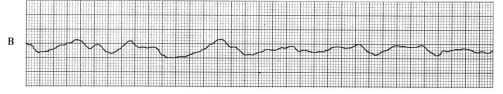

Fig. 8-28. A, Ventricular fibrillation with a coarse fibrillatory line. **B,** Ventricular fibrillation with a fine fibrillatory line.

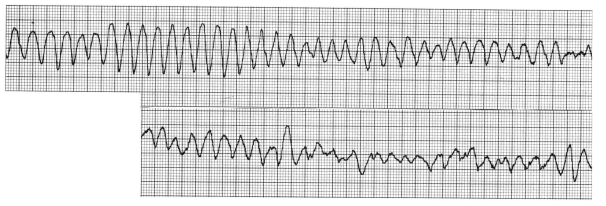

Fig. 8-29. Ventricular flutter and ventricular fibrillation.

in the ventricles and is easier to convert than a fine ventricular fibrillation (Fig. 8-28, *B*).

In Fig. 8-29 a very rapid ventricular tachycardia (ventricular flutter) deteriorates into ventricular fibrillation.

REENTRY: A CAUSE OF VENTRICULAR ECTOPICS

It is generally agreed that there are two mechanisms responsible for ventricular ectopic beats. One is *enhanced automaticity* of the His-Purkinje system due to an accelerated slow diastolic depolarization (phase 4). The other is *reentry* into the ventricular cell mass of a stimulus that should have been dissipated in its first passage. Reentry is due to depressed excitability and conductivity in isolated areas of the myocardium, which in turn create disunity in the repolarization process.

Both enhanced automaticity and reentry can be caused by the effect of catecholamines, ischemia, ionic imbalance, drugs, and stretch of the Purkinje fibers, as in congestive heart failure. The electrophysiology of reentry is as follows:

1 Ischemia reduces the resting membrane potential.
2 The action potential is directly dependent upon the resting membrane potential for its effectiveness (height and rate of rise).
3 As the resting membrane potential decreases (becomes less negative intracellularly), so do the slope and height of phase 0 (this relationship is referred to as "membrane responsiveness").
4 As the slope and height of the action potential falls, so does conduction velocity. This is known as *decremental conduction*.

Thus conduction can be markedly slowed in a group of ischemic cells, placing them out of phase with the rest of the ventricular myocardium, so that these cells are still refractory when the neighboring cells have become nonrefractory. A current then flows from the refractory (negative) area to the nonrefractory (positive) area, so that an impulse reenters the ventricles to generate an extrasystolic beat.

When, because of this decreased conductivity, an area of excitable tissue always exists, the impulse is propagated in a circular path. This movement of current is referred to as *circus reentry*. When this circular path does not exist, the reexcitation of the myocardium is called *focal reentry*.

PASSIVE ESCAPE MECHANISM OF THE VENTRICLES

When rhythmic impulses from the sinus node are no longer being transmitted into the ventricles, a lower pacemaker, usually in the bundle of His, will manifest its own inherent rhythm at a rate of 15 to 40 beats per minute. The ventricles will then be paced at this rate independently of the atria. This is a passive mechanism known as ventricular escape.

More specifically, ventricular complexes of normal configuration indicate

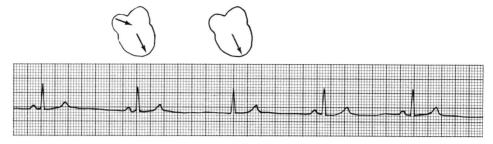

Fig. 8-30. Junctional escape due to sinus exit block.

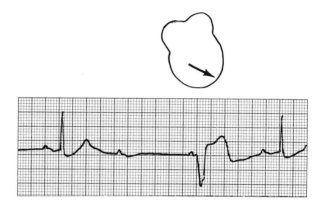

Fig. 8-31. Ventricular escape due to A-V conduction block.

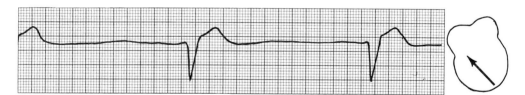

Fig. 8-32. Slow idioventricular rhythm.

that the pacemaker is above the bifurcation of the bundle of His and therefore the impulses are taking a normal path through the ventricles. This condition is called junctional escape. If the ventricular complexes are broad and the rate slower, it is evident that the pacemaker is below the bifurcation of the bundle of His. This condition is called ventricular escape.

Junctional escape

In Fig. 8-30 the bundle of His is seen to escape for one beat because of sinus bradycardia. The escape beat is of the same contour as the sinus-conducted beats because an impulse arising in the A-V junction will take a normal pathway in depolarizing the ventricles.

Notice that the R-R interval of both the sinus-conducted complex and the junctional escape beat is longer than the R-R intervals of the sinus-conducted complexes. This is the hallmark of the passive rhythm. It is not premature but late. It does not usurp control. It paces because the sinus node fails.

Ventricular escape

Fig. 8-31 depicts the failure of the sinus node to conduct impulses to the ventricle. After two nonconducted P waves there is ventricular escape. The escape beat is broad, indicating that the focus is below the bifurcation of the bundle of His.

Slow idioventricular rhythm

In Fig. 8-32 the ventricular rate is 23 and the QRS complexes are broad (0.20 second). This is evidence of a pacemaker low in the conductive system. P waves are not apparent. They may be seen in another lead, or they may be truly absent, in which case there is atrial standstill with an idioventricular rhythm.

SUMMARY

Ectopic foci in the ventricles usually originate in the His-Purkinje system. They may be either active or passive. An active focus depolarizes early, before it can be depolarized by the impulse from the sinus node. A passive focus depolarizes at its own rate when it is not depolarized early by an impulse from the sinus node. The location of the focus in the His-Purkinje system will determine the contour of the ectopic complex. If the focus is above the bifurcation of the bundle of His, the complex will be of normal contour. If the focus is below the bifurcation, the complex will be broad and distorted.

PVCs are serious, especially in the diseased heart. They are even more serious if they are frequent, multifocal, paired, and left ventricular or if they occur on the T wave. In ventricular tachycardia an ectopic focus completely dominates the ventricles. In ventricular fibrillation the cardiac contractions are ineffective because there is no unified electrical activity.

TEST TRACINGS

Before approaching the test tracings, recall what information you have already accumulated. First, look at the *rate* and determine if it is too fast, too slow, or normal. Is the rhythm regular? If so, you have already eliminated certain arrhythmias. Are there P waves? If so, are they regular and all of the same shape? Are the ventricular complexes regular and all of the same configuration?

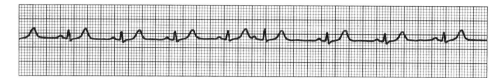

Fig. 8-33

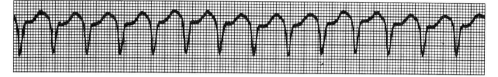

Fig. 8-34

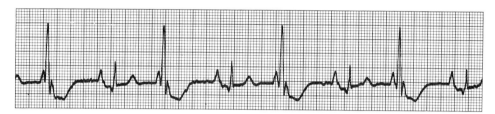

Fig. 8-35

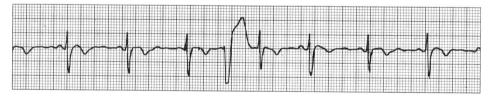

Fig. 8-36

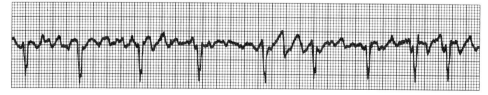

Fig. 8-37

ANSWERS

8-33 *PAC.* The single P' wave in this tracing immediately follows a T wave.

8-34 *Ventricular tachycardia.* The tracing consists of a continuous series of ventricular ectopic beats at a rate of 120.

8-35 *Ventricular bigeminy.* These bigeminal ventricular extrasystoles are end diastolic. The P wave preceding the aberrant beat is not premature, but the ventricular complex is.

8-36 *Interpolated PVC.* The basic sinus rate is 70. Therefore one would not expect an interpolated PVC. Although delayed, the normal ventricular response is not interrupted. There is also a wandering pacemaker. All of the P waves are not of the same shape. The flatter P waves are not premature but late. This is the hallmark of the wandering pacemaker that is a passive mechanism.

8-37 *Atrial fibrillation.* There is a very coarse fibrillatory line reflecting the lack of electrical unity in the fibrillating atria. If you felt that you saw P waves, look for this same contour before each QRS and remember that P' waves of atrial flutter repeat their pattern throughout the tracing.

9 The atrioventricular junction

The A-V junction is composed of the A-V node, bundle of His, and the bundle branches at their origins from the bundle of His (Fig. 9-1).

Impulses originating in the atria must travel this pathway in order to produce ventricular activation. Any defect in conduction across the A-V junction is known as heart block. The significance of the conduction defect depends upon the level of block within the A-V junction. This level is indicated by the width of the QRS complex. A broad QRS complex indicates involvement of the bundle branches. A normal QRS complex indicates that conduction is delayed in the A-V node or bundle of His.

INCIDENCE OF HEART BLOCK IN MYOCARDIAL INFARCTION

First-degree heart block is found in 7% to 10% of all patients with acute myocardial infarction, 5% will have second-degree heart block, and 5% to 6% will have complete heart block. This is usually a transient condition, and normal sinus rhythm will be restored within 2 weeks in 90% of patients.

FIRST-DEGREE A-V BLOCK

First-degree A-V block is a conduction defect of the A-V junction that manifests itself in a long P-R interval. The impulse from the sinus node is

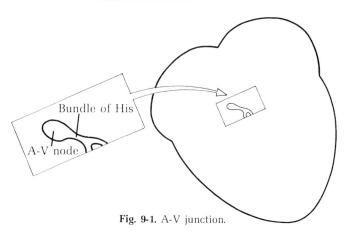

Fig. 9-1. A-V junction.

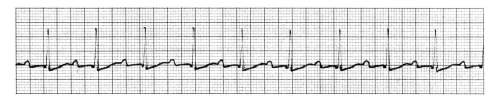

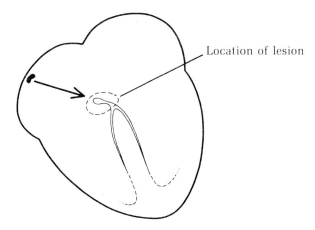

Fig. 9-2. Location of the conduction defect in first-degree heart block and tracing depicting narrow QRS.

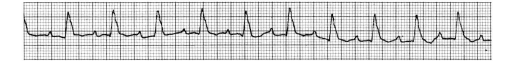

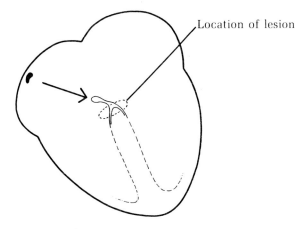

Fig. 9-3. Location of the conduction defect in first-degree heart block and tracing depicting broad QRS.

propagated in all beats but is delayed as it traverses the A-V junction (over 0.20 second).

In the tracing shown in Fig. 9-2 all P waves are conducted, but the P-R interval is too long (0.28 second). The QRS interval is not prolonged, indicating that the conduction delay is above the bifurcation of the bundle of His.

In Fig. 9-3 the P-R interval is too long (0.24 second), and the QRS interval is broadened (0.16 second), indicating that the lesion involves the bundle branches.

SECOND-DEGREE A-V BLOCK

Second-degree heart block is characterized by nonconducted P waves and is generally classified into two types: Mobitz type I (Wenckebach) and Mobitz type II.

Mobitz type I (Wenckebach)

Mobitz type I is characterized by the cyclic nonconduction of P waves that terminates a period of increasingly prolonged P-R intervals and shortening R-R intervals. The first R-R interval will be the longest of the group. The following R-R intervals will successively decrease or at least be shorter than the first. The QRS complexes are usually narrow since the conduction delay commonly occurs within the A-V node.

Fig. 9-4 shows the cyclic and gradual increase of the P-R interval until the last P wave of the group is not conducted. The first P-R interval beginning the cycle is 0.28 second. The second is 0.38 second and the third 0.40 second. The fourth P wave is not conducted. When three atrial complexes are conducted and one is not, the conduction ratio is said to be 4:3.

The gradual and progressive slowing of the impulse propagation seen in the Wenckebach phenomenon occurs within the A-V node. As the conduction velocity decreases, the refractory period lengthens, causing the P waves to fall closer and closer to this refractory period until it becomes inevitable that a P wave will eventually be nonconducted.

Of less common occurrence is the classic Mobitz type I phenomenon associated with broad QRS complexes, as seen in Fig. 9-5. The A-V conduction disturbance is thought to be at two levels. In the A-V node, conduction disturbance accounts for the increments in P-R intervals. In both bundle branches, it is reflected in the wide QRS.

Mobitz type II

In ECG tracings of Mobitz type II the nonconducted P wave is seen against a background of P-R intervals that are all the same. These intervals may or may not be prolonged. The QRS complexes are usually wide since the lesion most commonly involves both bundle branches.

Treatment and prognosis are governed by the level of the conduction delay within the A-V junction. A broadened QRS complex indicates a more

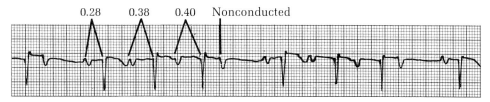

Fig. 9-4. Mobitz type I (Wenckebach) with a narrow QRS.

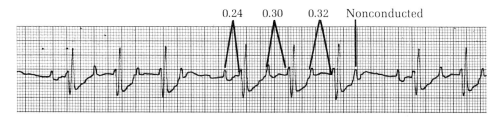

Fig. 9-5. Mobitz type I (Wenckebach) with a broad QRS.

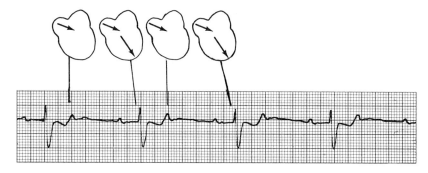

Fig. 9-6. Mobitz type II with 2:1 A-V conduction and a broad QRS.

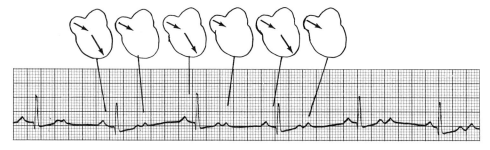

Fig. 9-7. Mobitz type II with 2:1 A-V conduction and a narrow QRS.

ominous anatomical lesion. In Fig. 9-6 there are two P waves for every QRS complex. The conduction ratio then is 2:1.

In some cases Mobitz type II A-V block is associated with normal QRS complexes. In Fig. 9-7 the P-R interval of the conducted beats is not prolonged (0.16 second).

COMPLETE HEART BLOCK

The sole muscular channel for the propagation of the electrical impulse from atria to ventricles is the A-V junction. If there is a lesion serious enough to block conduction at any level in the junction, complete A-V heart block results.

Complete heart block can result from lesions in one or more of the three sites illustrated in Fig. 9-8: the A-V node, the bundle of His, and the right and left bundle branches.

In complete heart block the rate and the dependability of the ventricular rhythm will be related to the level of the lesion in the A-V junction. A pacemaker at the top of the bundle of His will have a rate of about 50 and will be relatively dependable. However, if the pacemaker is lower in the A-V junction, at the branching segment of the bundle of His, the rate will be slower and less dependable.

The P waves in Fig. 9-9 can be seen to occur regularly at a rate of 100. They are totally independent of the ventricular rate of 46. The sinus node paces the atria, and the A-V junction paces the ventricles. Since the QRS complex is of normal duration (0.08 second), the ventricular pacemaker must be above the bifurcation of the bundle of His. This is called an *idiojunctional rhythm.*

The diagnosis of this arrhythmia is straightforward. "Walking out" the

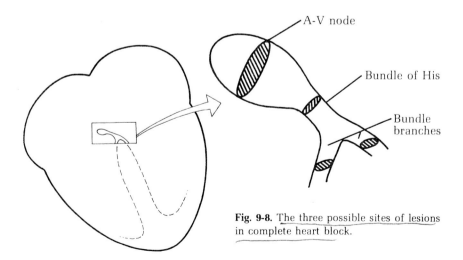

Fig. 9-8. The three possible sites of lesions in complete heart block.

P waves and R waves shows two independent pacemakers. In spite of this, an error is commonly made. After glancing briefly at the tracing, you might say that it is Mobitz type II with 2:1 A-V block, but if this were true, the P-R intervals of the conducted beats would all be the same.

The P waves occur at a rate of 75 in Fig. 9-10. They are regular and undisturbed by the ventricular rhythm of 36. This is complete heart block with an *idioventricular rhythm*. The broad QRS complex (0.12 second) indicates a focus below the branching of the bundle of His.

Fig. 9-11 shows complete heart block when the ventricular pacemaker fails, resulting in ventricular asystole.

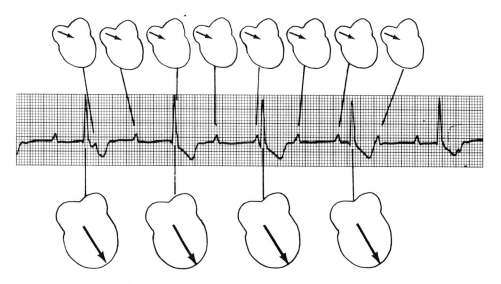

Fig. 9-9. Complete heart block with a junctional rhythm.

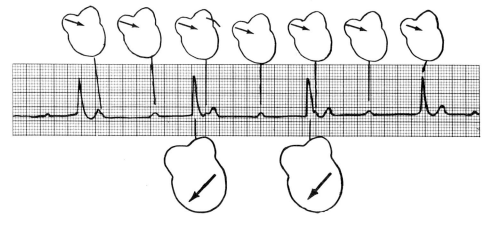

Fig. 9-10. Complete heart block with an idioventricular rhythm.

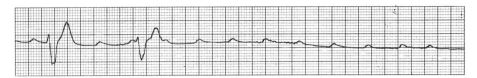

Fig. 9-11. Complete heart block with a failing ventricular pacemaker.

A-V JUNCTIONAL RHYTHMS

The shape of the P wave and the length of the P-R interval indicate whether a normal pacemaker is in command and whether A-V conduction is normal.

Historical background

In 1913 A. Zahn described what he called upper-, mid-, and low-nodal rhythms. This descriptive terminology was based on what was thought to be the level of the ectopic pacemaker in the A-V node. This conclusion was made because of the shape of the P' wave (inverted in leads II, III, and aV$_F$) and its relation to the QRS complex. If the inverted P' wave immediately preceded the QRS, and if a P'-R interval of less than 0.12 second was present, the focus was said to be in the upper region of the A-V node. If the P' wave was buried in the QRS, the focus was said to be centrally located within the A-V node. An inverted P' wave immediately following the QRS was said to originate from a focus in the lower region of the A-V node.

Today, through the use of the His bundle electrogram (HBE), it is known that the so-called "nodal" rhythms originate from a focus in the bundle of His. The A-V node itself does not have pacemaker cells. Its function is to delay impulses as they pass from atria to ventricles. Arrhythmias that involve automaticity, whether active or passive, will therefore be referred to as "junctional" rather than nodal. When the arrhythmia is caused by any aberration of the normal conduction through the A-V node, the term "nodal" will be used.

Whether the P' wave occurs before, during, or after the QRS complex is certainly a function of the relative speed of antegrade (forward) and retrograde (backward) conduction, irrespective of the level of the focus in the bundle of His. Since this level is not easily determined, it is more practical not to refer to it at all.

Active and passive junctional rhythms

Junctional rhythms are either active or passive. An active rhythm is due to an irritable A-V junction that takes command of the heart because of its rapid rate. Isolated premature junctional contractions are also active. Passive rhythms occur either because the sinus node fails or because it slows excessively. They are escape rhythms with a rate of between 40 and 60 beats per minute (the inherent rate of the A-V junction).

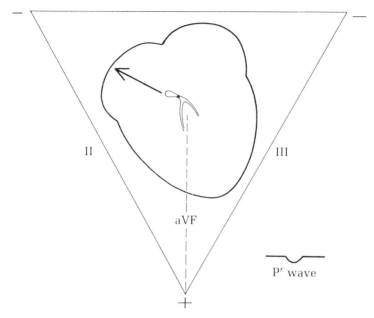

Fig. 9-12. Retrograde activation of the atria and the P′ wave in leads II, III, and aV_F.

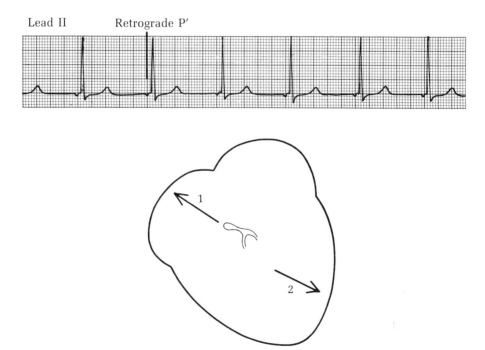

Fig. 9-13. Junctional rhythm—atrial activation precedes ventricular activation.

Lead II

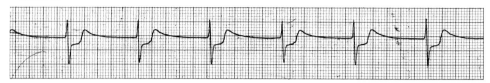

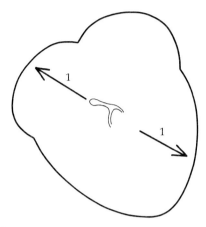

Fig. 9-14. Junctional rhythm—atrial and ventricular activation occur simultaneously.

Lead II

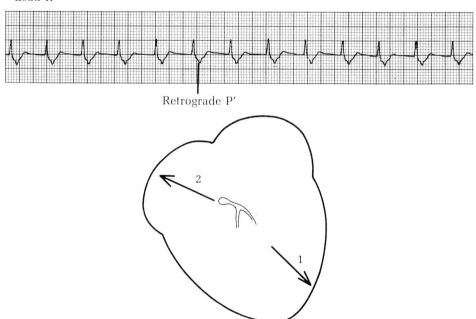

Retrograde P'

Fig. 9-15. Junctional rhythm (tachycardia)—ventricular activation precedes atrial activation.

Electrophysiology

If the A-V junctional region paces the heart, the P′ vector must travel in a retrograde direction in order to activate the atria. In leads II, III, and aV_F this current flows away from the positive terminal of these leads and causes a negative P′ wave to be recorded, as shown in Fig. 9-12.

An inverted P′ wave that is apparent shortly before the QRS complex indicates that atrial activation took place in a retrograde direction, immediately preceding ventricular activation.

At a rate of 58 the tracing in Fig. 9-13 is a junctional bradycardia (a passive rhythm). The inverted P′ wave and the short P′-R interval (0.08 second) indicate a junctional focus. If the P′-R interval exceeds 0.11 second, the focus is considered to be on the floor of the right atrium.

In Fig. 9-14 there are no apparent P waves. The ventricular rhythm is regular at a rate of 57. Atrial depolarization and ventricular depolarization are accomplished simultaneously, causing the P′ wave to be hidden within the QRS complex.

The rhythm is passive since a normal sinus node would be in command at a rate above 60. Thus the A-V junction is pacing the heart at its own inherent rate of 57 because the sinus node has failed in its function.

In Fig. 9-15 a P′ wave is apparent immediately following the QRS complex. This indicates that retrograde depolarization of the atria has occurred immediately following depolarization of the ventricles. The pacemaker is located in the bundle of His, and there is a more delayed retrograde conduction to the atria than is seen in Figs. 9-13 and 9-14. Since the rate is 120, this is an active rhythm. An irritable A-V junction is usurping control.

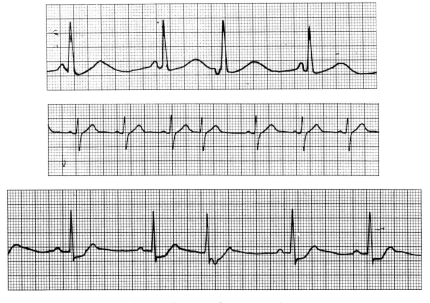

Fig. 9-16. Junctional premature beats.

PREMATURE JUNCTIONAL CONTRACTION

The A-V junction may also generate an isolated premature stimulus. The hallmarks of this arrhythmia are the same as those of the junctional rhythms. The P' wave will be either just before, within, or after the QRS complex and will be inverted in leads II, III, and aV$_F$. Since the sinus node will be depolarized early because of this ectopic stimulus, there will not be a full compensatory pause (Fig. 9-16).

SUMMARY

Conduction defects of the A-V junction cause heart block. The duration of the QRS complex indicates the level of the conduction delay within the A-V junction.

In first-degree A-V block the P-R interval is prolonged beyond 0.20 second. In second-degree A-V block the P-R interval may be either normal or prolonged, but some impulses are not propagated. In complete heart block the atria and ventricles beat separately. The atria are usually paced by the sinus node at a normal rate, and the ventricles are paced by the His-Purkinje system. A pacemaker above the bifurcation of the bundle of His produces what is called an idiojunctional rhythm. A pacemaker below the bundle of His produces an idioventricular rhythm. The rate of the ventricular pacemaker in complete heart block is usually not above 40 beats per minute.

The A-V junctional tissue is usually dominated by the more rapidly beating sinus node. It may become the pacemaker if it depolarizes more rapidly than the sinus node (an active rhythm) or if the sinus node fails in its function (a passive rhythm). Isolated premature junctional beats may also occur.

TEST TRACINGS

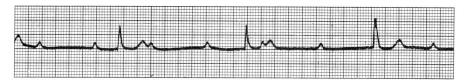

Fig. 9-17

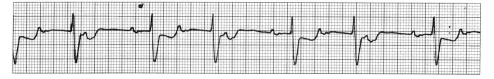

Fig. 9-18

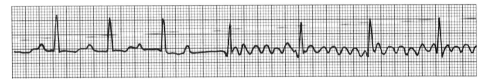

Fig. 9-19

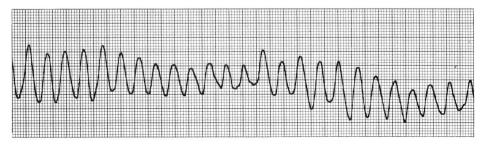

Fig. 9-20

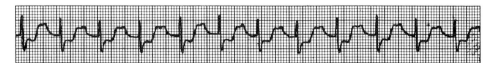

Fig. 9-21

ANSWERS

9-17 *Complete heart block.* The P waves are clearly seen and occur regularly at a rate of 72. The ventricles are beating independently under the control of a nodal pacemaker at a rate of 32.

9-18 *Mobitz type I.* The first P-R interval of each group is 0.28 second. The second P-R interval is 0.48 second, and the third P wave falls on the T wave and is not conducted. This is the cyclic prolongation of the P-R interval that describes Mobitz type I (Wenckebach phenomenon). The QRS interval is also prolonged, indicating that there are lesions at two levels in the A-V junction: at the A-V node and at the bifurcation of the bundle of His.

9-19 *Mobitz type I followed by a junctional rhythm and atrial flutter with 6:1 and 7:1 A-V conduction.* In the first part of the strip the P-R interval gradually increases from 0.20 to 0.36 second, until finally there is nonconduction. The A-V junction then begins to pace the ventricles at a rate of 57. Notice that the A-V junctional complex is slightly different from the sinus-conducted beats. After the first junctional complex, one can see the typical sawtooth pattern of atrial flutter, in which the atrial rate varies from 325 to 400 beats per minute. Because the A-V junction is pacing the heart independently of the atrial ectopic rhythm, the ventricular complexes have no constant relationship to the flutter waves. (See Fig. 7-13.)

9-20 *Ventricular flutter.* The ventricular rate is 225, and the complexes have become rounded and are no longer angular.

9-21 *First-degree A-V block.* The P-R interval is 0.24 second. All impulses are conducted, but conduction is delayed. Sinus tachycardia is also present.

10 Bundle branch block

One of the most distinctive examples of an intraventricular conduction defect is the obstruction of impulse conduction in one of the bundle branches.

Ordinarily the two lateral walls of the ventricles depolarize at almost the same time (Fig. 10-1). The current reaches both bundles at the same time, and the entire ventricular muscle is depolarized.

An obstruction in either of the bundle branches would cause the affected side to be depolarized late (Fig. 10-2). This delay in the process of depolarization and deviation of the ventricular vector results in a distorted QRS complex of more than 0.10 second in duration in right bundle branch block and more than 0.11 second in left bundle branch block.

NORMAL VENTRICULAR ACTIVATION TIME (VAT)

The length of time required for the depolarization wave to travel from the endocardium to the epicardium is called the ventricular activation time, or VAT. It will normally reach its peak in the left ventricle because the left ventricle is larger and takes longer to depolarize than the right ventricle.

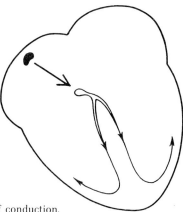

Fig. 10-1. Normal pathway of conduction.

The VAT is measured from the Q wave, or first evidence of ventricular depolarization, to the peak of the R wave (Fig. 10-3).

VAT in left ventricular leads (V₅ and V₆)

In leads facing the left ventricle the peak of the R wave occurs in 0.04 second or less.

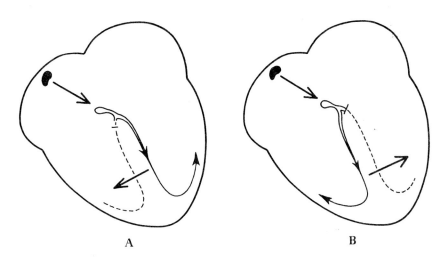

Fig. 10-2. A, Right bundle branch block (RBBB). **B,** Left bundle branch block (LBBB).

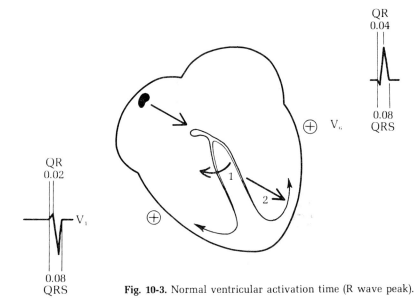

Fig. 10-3. Normal ventricular activation time (R wave peak).

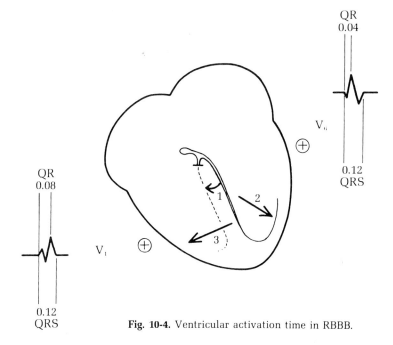

Fig. 10-4. Ventricular activation time in RBBB.

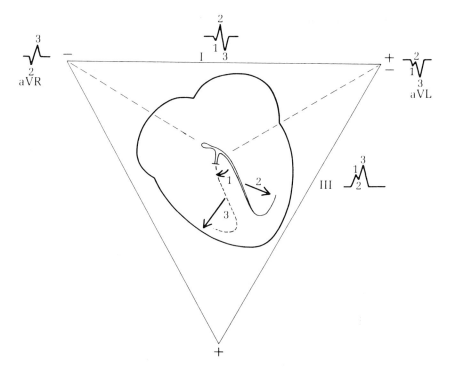

Fig. 10-5. RBBB. Electrical events as seen in leads I, III, aV_L, and aV_R.

VAT in right ventricular leads (V₁ and V₂)

In leads facing the right ventricle the R wave represents only interventricular (I-V) septal activation and occurs in 0.02 second or less.

RIGHT BUNDLE BRANCH BLOCK (RBBB)

When the impulse is blocked in the right bundle branch, the left ventricle is activated normally, and the right ventricle is activated late through the I-V septum instead of through the accelerated Purkinje network.

Right ventricular leads (V₁ and V₂) and the VAT in RBBB

Because of the block in conduction through the right bundle branch, the right ventricle will be activated last. This delayed vector will originate in the unaffected left side and will flow into the positive electrode of V_1, causing a broad terminal R′ wave. The VAT is markedly delayed (0.08 second), as shown in Fig. 10-4.

Left ventricular leads (V₅ and V₆) and the VAT in RBBB

Since the left ventricle is activated normally, the leads facing this ventricle will have a normal VAT (R wave peak) (Fig. 10-4).

QRS complex in RBBB

The terminal deflections of the QRS complex are the clue to the diagnosis of RBBB. The abnormal late depolarization of the right ventricle is reflected in these final deflections. The main ECG features are as follows:

1 A prolonged QRS duration (0.11 second or more)
2 Notched deflections in V_1 (rSR′)
3 T wave changes
4 Peak of R wave (VAT) markedly delayed in right ventricular leads (V_1) and normal in left ventricular leads (V_6)

Electrical events as seen in V₁ and V₆ (RBBB)

	V₁	V₆
1 Normal septal activation from left to right	Small r wave	Small q wave
2 Normal large left ventricular vector	S wave	R wave
3 Delayed depolarization of right ventricle	Wide terminal R′ wave	Wide terminal S wave

Electrical events as seen in unipolar and standard limb leads (RBBB)

Because the limb leads are affected by the position of the heart, they alone are not reliable criteria for a diagnosis of bundle branch block. They do, however, show characteristic features (Fig. 10-5):

Leads I and aV_L	Terminal broad S wave
Leads III and aV_R	Terminal broad R′ wave

LEFT BUNDLE BRANCH BLOCK (LBBB)

Before continuing, it is suggested that at this point you attempt to draw the wave deflections of LBBB for yourself.

1 Draw the heart and the conductive system.

2 Indicate a block in the left bundle branch and construct the resultant ventricular vectors.

3 Indicate the electrodes of V_1 and V_6.

4 Draw the ECG.

Recall that vector flow toward a positive terminal will cause a positive deflection, and vector flow away from a positive terminal will cause a negative deflection. The strength of the vector will determine the amplitude of the deflection.

Right ventricular leads (V_1 and V_2) and the VAT in LBBB

The right ventricle is activated normally. Therefore leads facing this ventricle will have a normal VAT (0.02 second), as shown in Fig. 10-6.

Left ventricular leads (V_5 and V_6) and the VAT in LBBB

Since the impulse is blocked in the left bundle branch, the left ventricle will be activated late by a vector from the I-V septum instead of via the accelerated pathway of the Purkinje network. Leads facing the left ventricle will therefore have a delayed VAT (more than 0.06 second), as shown in Fig. 10-6.

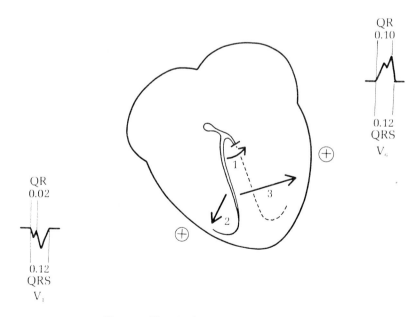

Fig. 10-6. Ventricular activation time in LBBB.

QRS complex in LBBB

The terminal deflections of the QRS complex that reflect the late depolarization of the left ventricle are the clue to diagnosis. The main ECG features are as follows:

1 A prolonged QRS interval (0.12 second or more)
2 Notched deflections in V_6 ("M" slurred complex)
3 T wave changes
4 Peak of R wave (VAT) markedly delayed in left ventricular leads (V_6) and normal in right ventricular leads (V_1)

Electrical events as seen in V₁ and V₆ (LBBB)

		V_1	V_6
1	Abnormal septal activation from right to left	Small q wave	Small r wave
2	Normal small right ventricular vector	Small upward deflection	Small downward deflection
3	Delayed depolarization of left ventricle	Wide terminal S wave	Wide terminal R' wave

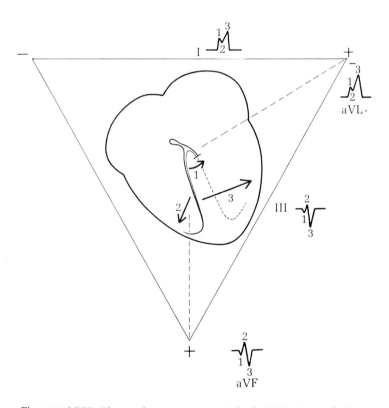

Fig. 10-7. LBBB. Electrical events as seen in leads I, III, aV_L, and aV_F.

Electrical events as seen in unipolar and standard limb leads (LBBB)

The limb leads are affected by the position of the heart. They alone are therefore not reliable criteria for a diagnosis of LBBB. They do, however, show characteristic features (Fig. 10-7):

Leads I and aV$_L$	Wide slurred R wave
Leads III and aV$_F$	Wide S wave

INCOMPLETE RBBB

If the right bundle branch is only partially blocked, the impulse will enter the right ventricle through the normal His-Purkinje pathway. However, it will be delayed at the site of the block, causing late activation of the right ventricle. This late right ventricular vector is also seen in complete RBBB. Therefore the components of the ventricular complex will be the same. The QRS interval, however, will be less than 0.11 second.

INCOMPLETE LBBB

Partial blockage of the left bundle branch will delay the transmission of the impulse through the bundle. The right ventricle will be depolarized first with a right-to-left current across the I-V septum. The QRS interval will be less than 0.12 second. The diagnosis is therefore made because of the initial right ventricular forces that will be the same as those seen in complete LBBB.

The differential diagnosis is sometimes difficult since the QRS resembles that seen in left ventricular hypertrophy.

HEMIBLOCK

The three main terminal fascicles (bundles) of the intraventricular conduction system are the right bundle branch and the anterior and posterior divisions of the left bundle branch (Fig. 10-8).

When conduction is blocked in either fascicle of the left bundle branch, the condition is referred to as hemiblock: left anterior hemiblock (LAH) or left posterior hemiblock (LPH).

Conduction may be permanently or only intermittently interrupted in one (unifascicular block), two (bifascicular block), or all three (trifascicular block) fascicles. Frequently complete A-V block is preceded by the presence of RBBB plus LAH. The anterior division of the left bundle branch has the same anatomical origin as the right bundle branch (Fig. 10-8). Thus a small lesion may injure both of these fascicles.

Left anterior hemiblock (LAH)

The main blood supply to the anterior division of the left bundle branch comes from the left coronary artery; hence LAH is often seen in anterolateral and anteroseptal myocardial infarction. Because the initial vectors are inferior

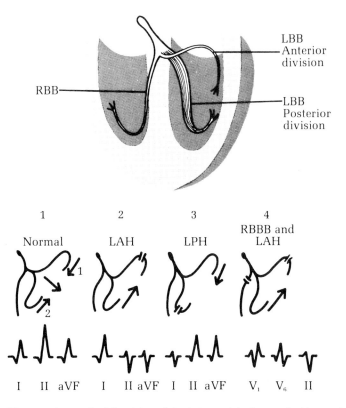

Fig. 10-8. Three main terminal fascicles of the intraventricular conduction system.

and to the right (depolarization of the septum), there will be a small r wave in leads II, III, and aV_F and a small q wave in lead I. Because the left ventricle is activated through the posterior division of the left bundle branch (Fig. 10-8), there will be a marked left axis deviation (greater than −60 degrees) and deep S waves in leads II, III, and aV_F.

Left anterior hemiblock (LAH) and RBBB

If RBBB is accompanied by a left axis deviation of greater than −60 degrees, LAH is suspected to coexist.

The initial ventricular forces are caused by the hemiblock and will determine the direction of the mean QRS axis. The terminal forces are caused by the RBBB. The initial forces will cause, as in pure LAH, a small r wave in leads II, III, and aV_F, a small q wave in lead I, and S waves in leads II, III, and aV_F.

The late activation of the right ventricle due to the RBBB is best seen in lead V_1, which has a broad terminal R wave, and in lead V_6, which has a broad terminal S wave.

Left posterior hemiblock (LPH) and RBBB

Block of the posterior division of the left bundle branch is uncommon since it is less vulnerable due to its thickness, length, position, and dual blood supply (right and left coronary arteries). LPH is almost always associated with RBBB. The ECG will manifest a right axis deviation of +120 degrees.

The initial ventricular forces are caused by the LPH and will determine the direction of the mean QRS axis. The terminal forces are caused by the RBBB.

Initially the left ventricle is activated through the anterior division of the left bundle branch, causing a small q wave in leads II, III, and aV_F and a small r wave in lead I. Because the posterior wall of the left ventricle and the right ventricular wall are on the same plane, the delayed activation of the posterior wall of the left ventricle (LPH) and the late activation of the right ventricle (RBBB) cause an S wave in lead I and R waves in leads II, III, and aV_F.

SUMMARY

Right and left bundle branch blocks are distinctive intraventricular conduction defects. The most significant ECG feature of each is the late activation of the affected ventricle. This is most easily recognized in the right and left precordial leads since the limb leads are affected by the heart position.

The conductive system of the heart is trifascicular in structure. The left bundle branch has two divisions (anterior and posterior). A block of the anterior division is termed left anterior hemiblock, and a block of the posterior division is termed left posterior hemiblock. LAH and RBBB often coexist, and as a precursor of symptomatic A-V block take on important diagnostic significance.

TEST TRACINGS

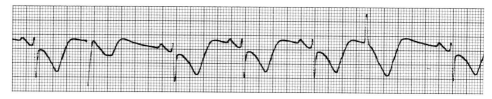

Fig. 10-9

Lead II

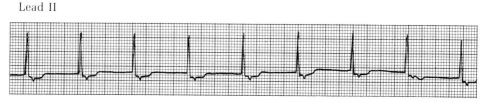

Fig. 10-10

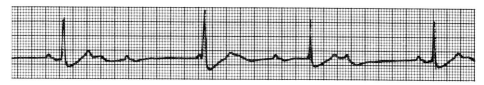

Fig. 10-11

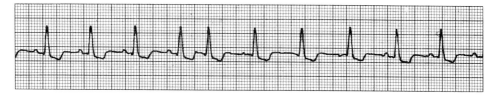

Fig. 10-12

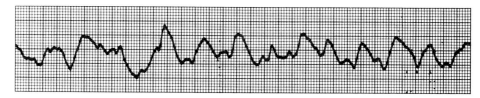

Fig. 10-13

ANSWERS

10-9 *Sinus bradycardia with septal, bifocal PVCs.* The basic rate is 58. The PVCs are of two different configurations, indicating two ectopic foci. Neither PVC is over 0.08 second in duration. There are therefore two foci in the I-V septum.

10-10 *A junctional rhythm.* In lead II a negative P' wave indicates a focus low in the atrium. If the P' wave follows the QRS, the pacemaker is located in the A-V junction and delayed retrograde conduction is present.

10-11 *Mobitz type II with junctional escape.* At first glance this might appear to be a complete heart block. The ventricular rhythm, however, is irregular, and this should tell you to look for ventricular capture and junctional escape. The first and last complexes are conducted and have the same P-R interval. The second ventricular complex is an escape beat because the P wave is too close to conduct. The third R wave may or may not have been conducted.

10-12 *Wandering pacemaker.* The first premature beat is a PAC followed by three complexes (passive) from different foci in the atrium and A-V junction.

10-13 *Ventricular fibrillation.* Chaotic ventricular activity is reflected in this erratic ECG pattern.

11 Aberrant ventricular conduction

Aberrant means straying from the right way or wandering. In electrocardiography the term is used to indicate that although an impulse may have entered the ventricle in the normal way through the A-V node and bundle of His, its pathway within the ventricles is errant. Although bundle branch block and some ectopic ventricular impulses fit this description, the term applies only to the transient conduction defect.

Aberrant ventricular conduction occurs most often when, because of rapid rates, very premature atrial contractions, and/or changes in cycle length, the His-Purkinje system is not completely repolarized and is therefore functionally unable to conduct normally. In addition to incomplete repolarization, aberrancy may also be due to a reduction in the membrane potential and/or to a reduction in the rate of rise of phase 0 of the action potential (membrane responsiveness).

Because the right bundle branch repolarizes slightly later than the left bundle branch, it is more susceptible to block. This is the pattern (RBBB) most often assumed by the aberrant ventricular impulse (Fig. 11-1).

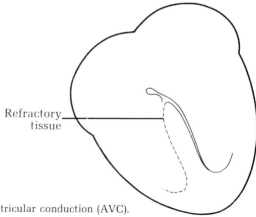

Refractory tissue

Fig. 11-1. Aberrant ventricular conduction (AVC).

PREMATURE ATRIAL CONTRACTIONS (PACs) AND ABERRANT VENTRICULAR CONDUCTION (AVC)

AVC following a PAC is commonly mistaken for a premature ventricular contraction (PVC), especially when the P′ wave is hidden in the preceding T wave. A less than full compensatory pause should alert you to examine the preceding T wave more carefully for signs of a premature atrial beat. Occasionally, however, a full compensatory pause will follow the PAC because an ectopic stimulus in the atria may suppress the sinus node pacemaker. Suppression of the sinus node may delay the next impulse long enough for it to occur at the normal time.

The premature complex shown in Fig. 11-2 looks, at first glance, like a PVC. However, there is not a full compensatory pause and, after close examination, a P′ wave can be seen on the preceding T wave. This is a PAC with AVC.

At a rate of 48 the tracing in Fig. 11-2 also represents sinus bradycardia. When the ventricular rate decreases, the time taken for the repolarization process lengthens. It is therefore more likely that a premature atrial stimulus will meet with refractory tissue when the dominant rate is slow. The coupling interval is, of course, also a factor. The closer the PAC is to the preceding ventricular complex, the more inevitable is aberration. Both a lengthened action potential due to bradycardia and a short coupling interval are causative factors in the AVC shown in Fig. 11-2.

POSTEXTRASYSTOLIC BEAT AND AVC

Because of the change in cycle length, the beat following the ventricular extrasystole is often aberrant in both the QRS and the T wave.

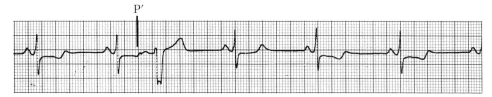

Fig. 11-2. Premature atrial contraction (PAC) with AVC.

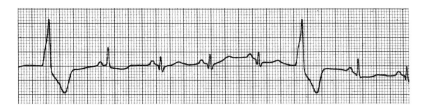

Fig. 11-3. AVC of a postextrasystolic beat.

In Fig. 11-3 both T wave and QRS changes are seen in the complex following the ventricular extrasystole. Because of a shortening of the previous cycle (PVC), the action potential shortened to accommodate a faster rate. The resultant ECG complex is sometimes aberrant.

ATRIAL FIBRILLATION AND AVC

Unless a His bundle electrogram (HBE) is taken it is impossible to determine whether the aberrant-looking complexes sometimes seen in atrial fibrillation are ventricular ectopic in origin or whether they are produced by aberrant conduction of the erratic supraventricular activity. Aberration is, however, more likely to be present when there is a short R-R interval that has been preceded by a long R-R interval (Fig. 11-4). Since lengthening of the cycle causes the repolarization time to lengthen also, immediate shortening of the cycle may cause the stimulus to meet with refractory tissue—an occurrence sometimes referred to as Ashman's phenomenon.

SUPRAVENTRICULAR TACHYCARDIA AND AVC

When the ventricular rate suddenly becomes more rapid, the repolarization time does not change suddenly. Rather, there is a gradual adjustment. The suddenly accelerated stimulus will in some cases meet with incompletely repolarized tissue in the His-Purkinje system and result in aberrant ventricular complexes. A classic example of this is shown in Fig. 11-5.

DIFFERENTIAL DIAGNOSIS OF SUPRAVENTRICULAR TACHYCARDIA

It is often impossible to differentiate electrocardiographically between supraventricular tachycardia with AVC and ventricular tachycardia. There are only a few signs that are conclusive and they are not always seen. A diagnosis can more easily be made if the following are seen: the onset of the tachycardia, isolated extrasystoles, visible P waves, Dressler beats, and right bundle branch block (RBBB) pattern in the aberrant complex.

Onset of the tachycardia

A premature P′ wave will be seen preceding a supraventricular tachycardia (Fig. 11-5). A premature ventricular beat will be seen preceding a ventricular tachycardia. Such is the case in Fig. 11-6, where the ventricular tachycardia is accompanied by retrograde conduction to the atria with each alternate beat (2:1 retrograde conduction).

Isolated extrasystoles

A diagnosis of supraventricular tachycardia with AVC would be reasonably certain if an AVC complex of the same contour as the tachycardia were seen in a preceding isolated complex. By the same token, a diagnosis of ventricular tachycardia would be certain if an isolated PVC of the same contour as the tachycardia were seen in a previous tracing.

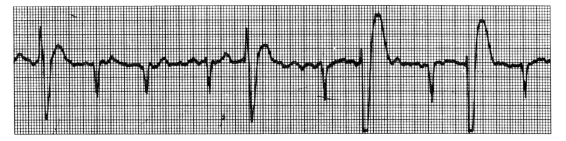

Fig. 11-4. Atrial fibrillation and AVC versus ventricular ectopic beats.

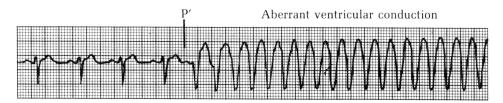

Fig. 11-5. Onset of atrial tachycardia with AVC.

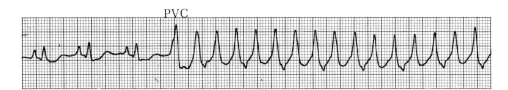

Fig. 11-6. Onset of ventricular tachycardia.

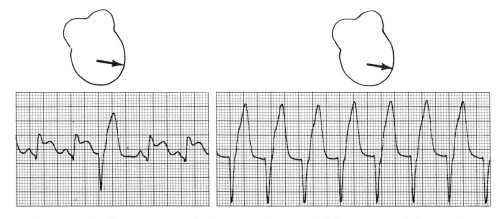

Fig. 11-7. Isolated premature ventricular contraction (PVC) of the same morphology as the ventricular tachycardia.

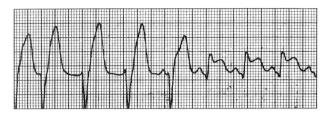

Fig. 11-8. Positive signs of dissociation.

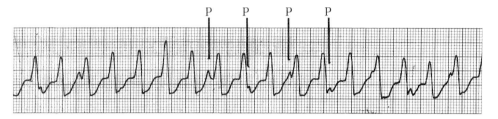

Fig. 11-9. Sign of dissociation in ventricular tachycardia.

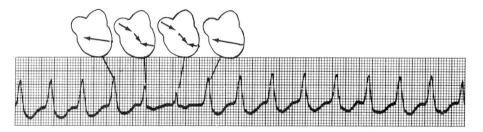

Fig. 11-10. Ventricular tachycardia with Dressler beats (ventricular fusion).

For example, a previous tracing of this patient (Fig. 11-7) shows an isolated septal PVC of the same morphology as the tachycardia. Certainly a ventricular tachycardia with narrow complexes of septal origin would easily have been mistaken for a supraventricular tachycardia had the isolated PVC not been seen (Fig. 11-8).

As the tachycardia terminates, positive signs of dissociation are seen. The P wave begins to emerge from the QRS, and finally there is a ventricular fusion beat (partial capture). The sinus node again assumes control at a rate of 100.

Visible P waves

Independent P waves that are dissociated from ventricular activity are conclusive evidence of ventricular tachycardia (Fig. 11-9).

Conversely, if an ectopic P′ wave is seen in relation to each AVC, a diagnosis of supraventricular tachycardia cannot always be made since this

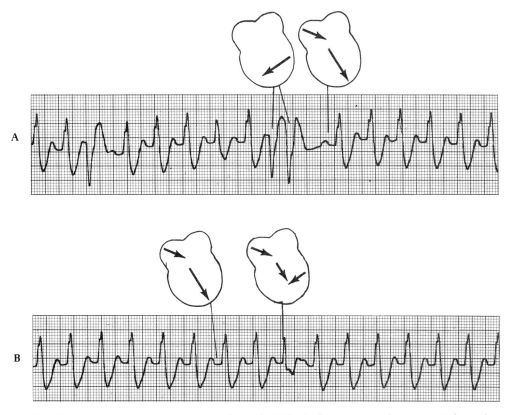

Fig. 11-11. A, Supraventricular tachycardia with PVCs. **B,** Same patient. Supraventricular tachycardia with Dressler or ventricular fusion beats.

relationship may also be seen in ventricular tachycardia with 1:1 retrograde conduction. However, if the P′ wave is upright in lead II, one would be safe in assuming that the pacemaker was in the atrium and that impulses were being conducted to the ventricle.

Dressler beats

Narrower beats of lesser amplitude, such as those seen in Fig. 11-10, are due to ventricular fusion and are termed Dressler beats.

Dressler beats are suggestive of but not diagnostic of dissociation and ventricular tachycardia. They are not diagnostic since they may also occur in a supraventricular tachycardia. These narrow beats represent the complete or partial capture of the ventricles by the independently beating atria.

In Fig. 11-11, *B,* the narrower complex that interrupts the series of broad, tall ventricular complexes is a ventricular fusion beat. In this case, however, it is caused by a ventricular ectopic vector fusing with a sinus-conducted impulse. In the first tracing (Fig. 11-11, *A*) the complexes from both foci can be seen. The coupled PVCs are followed by a compensatory pause that allows us to see the sinus P wave and its ventricular response. This ventricular response manifests the same QRS contour as is seen in the tachycardia. Therefore there is no doubt that the tachycardia is supraventricular (sinus) in origin; yet there is a Dressler beat.

Right bundle branch block (RBBB) pattern

Since this is the pattern most often assumed by the aberrantly conducted ventricular complex, its presence would be indicative of supraventricular tachycardia with AVC.

SUMMARY

Ventricular aberration will occur if the ventricle is still partially refractory at the time of the next stimulus. The term "AVC" is reserved for the occasional errant pathway that a supraventricular stimulus takes through the ventricle and applies only to a transient conduction defect.

PACs with AVC are frequently misdiagnosed as PVCs. Look for the premature P′ wave hidden in the T. Measure the compensatory pause. Differentiating between supraventricular tachycardia and ventricular tachycardia is often impossible with the ECG alone. There are a few clues:

1 Look for P waves. Independent P waves are diagnostic of dissociation and ventricular tachycardia. However, P′ waves associated with each ventricular complex are indicative but not diagnostic of supraventricular tachycardia.

2 Look for Dressler beats. These narrower beats of lesser amplitude are strongly suggestive of dissociation. They are, however, seldom seen in the tachycardias with a rate of over 150.

3 Look for isolated extrasystoles in a previous tracing. A PAC with AVC of the same contour as the tachycardia is an almost certain indication that the arrhythmia is supraventricular in origin. By the same token, a PVC of the same contour as the tachycardia would support a diagnosis of ventricular tachycardia.

4 Look at the onset of the tachycardia. A PAC would begin a supraventricular tachycardia. A PVC would begin a ventricular tachycardia.

TEST TRACINGS

Lead II

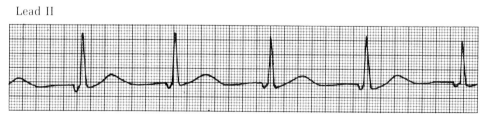

Fig. 11-12

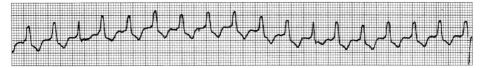

Fig. 11-13

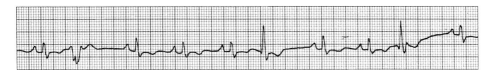

Fig. 11-14

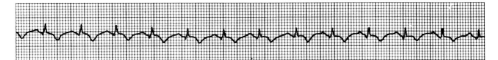

Fig. 11-15

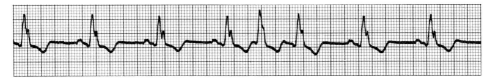

Fig. 11-16

ANSWERS

11-12 *Junctional bradycardia.* At a rate of 43 this is a passive escape rhythm. In lead II a negative P′ wave indicates retrograde conduction. The short P′-R interval (0.08 second) indicates that the focus is below the A-V node.

11-13 *Ventricular tachycardia.* The rate of this tachycardia is 140. There are two Dressler beats visible. These two factors are very suggestive of a diagnosis of ventricular tachycardia.

11-14 *Bifocal PVCs.* The basic rhythm is sinus conducted, and the rate is 75. The PVCs are of two different forms, indicating two foci in the ventricles.

11-15 *Sinus tachycardia.* The rate is 122. Normal P waves are visible before each QRS complex.

11-16 *Bundle branch block with an interpolated PVC.* The sinus-conducted QRS complexes are broad and notched. A PVC occurs without interrupting the regular sinus-conducted complexes (interpolated). The P-R interval of this post-extrasystolic beat is prolonged.

12 Preexcitation

Normally there is a delay of impulse conduction through the A-V junction to allow for ventricular filling. If ventricular depolarization occurs earlier than it would had the impulse traveled via the normal conduction pathway, preexcitation is said to exist. In this chapter we will discuss the accelerated conduction caused by the bundle of Kent and by the James bundle.

WOLFF-PARKINSON-WHITE (WPW) SYNDROME

Recent studies support the theory that it is possible for preexcitation to occur only if there is an additional muscular connection (muscle bundle) between the atrium and the ventricle. The muscle bundle that is present in Wolff-Parkinson-White (WPW) syndrome is called the bundle of Kent. It is thought to be an extension of the atrioventricular myocardium rather than a specialized conductive tissue.

Electrophysiology

Premature ventricular excitation via this accessory bundle would cause a short P-R interval and a prolonged ventricular conduction time (QRS interval). This premature excitation would also cause a small-amplitude heavy slurring of the first part of the ventricular complex. This premature component of the QRS complex is called the *delta* wave.

ECG changes

1 *P-R intervals:* 0.11 second or less (P-R segment absent)
2 *QRS duration:* 0.12 second or more
3 *Delta wave* (slurring of the upstroke or downstroke of the main ventricular deflection)

Anatomical aspects

WPW syndrome is divided into type A and type B. In both types a distinctive ECG and a history of paroxysmal tachycardias are the diagnostic features.

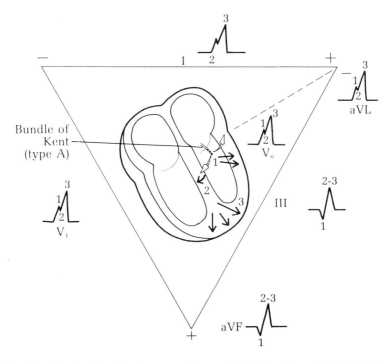

Fig. 12-1. Bundle of Kent and ventricular vectors in type A Wolff-Parkinson-White (WPW) syndrome.

Type A

It is thought that in type A WPW syndrome the bundle of Kent connects the left atrium with the left ventricular epicardium (posterior) (Fig. 12-1).

The delta wave is thought to be caused by the excitation of the ventricular tissue at the termination of the bundle of Kent (epicardial) and the resultant intramural vector that travels from the posterior epicardium to the endocardium (anteriorly). This early ventricular activation is therefore in an anterior and either a superior or inferior direction.

Thus the delta wave in leads I, aV_L, V_1, and V_6 will be positive. There will be a Q or QS wave in leads III and aV_F (Fig. 12-2).

Type B

In type B WPW syndrome the bundle of Kent connects the right atrium with the right ventricle. It is thought that this anomalous bundle terminates in the epicardium of the anterolateral aspect of the right ventricle. The right ventricle would then depolarize first by an excitation wave across the ventricular surface. The left ventricle would depolarize in a normal manner, being activated through the A-V junction (Fig. 12-3).

The delta wave is thought to be caused by the abnormal right ventric-

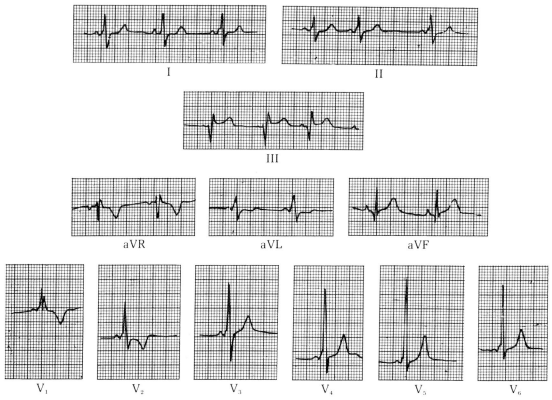

Fig. 12-2. Twelve-lead ECG. Type A WPW syndrome. (Courtesy Dr. Robert Braun.)

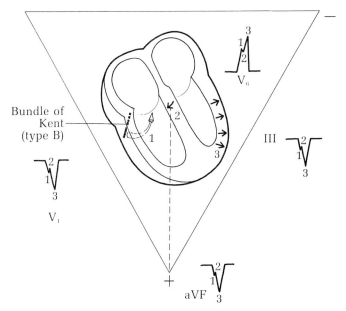

Fig. 12-3. Bundle of Kent and ventricular vectors in type B WPW syndrome.

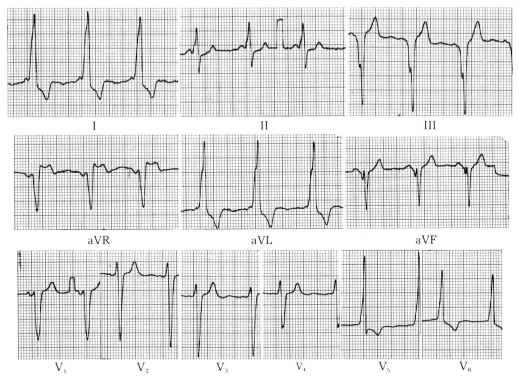

Fig. 12-4. Twelve-lead ECG. Type B WPW syndrome. (Courtesy Dr. Burton W. Fink.)

ular excitation process, proceeding from the termination of the bundle of Kent posteriorly and to the left.

These initial electrical forces would be reflected in V_1 as a QS, an rS, or a biphasic delta wave and in V_6 as a positive delta wave and a tall R. Q or QS waves are frequently seen in leads III and aV_F (Fig. 12-4).

It has been suggested that the characteristic QRS complex of type B WPW syndrome is due to a fusion beat resulting from the collision of forces from the early activation of the right ventricle and normal activation of the left ventricle. Note the opposing vectors 1 and 2 in Fig. 12-3.

Supraventricular tachycardia and WPW syndrome

Supraventricular tachycardias are often seen in patients with WPW conduction. They are said to be due to a retrograde atrial excitation that is attributed to a circular movement of the depolarization wave from the atrium across the A-V junction and back again to the atrium via the then nonrefractory bundle of Kent (reentry) (Fig. 12-5).

Since the bundle of Kent depolarizes first, it is nonrefractory while the ventricle is still being activated. A return of the impulse to the atrium via

Lead II

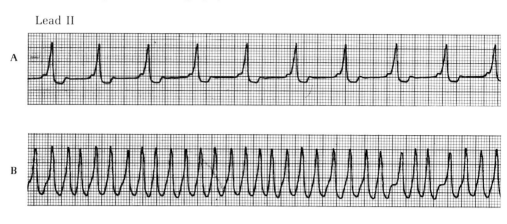

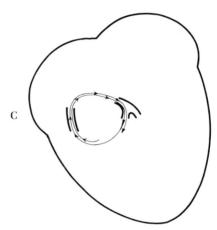

Fig. 12-5. A, WPW syndrome. **B,** Supraventricular tachycardia. **C,** Path of reentry into the atria via the bundle of Kent.

this accessory pathway is then possible, and a reciprocal rhythm is thus established.

The two tracings in Fig. 12-5 are from the same patient. The first tracing shows the short P-R and broad QRS of WPW syndrome. The second tracing shows a supraventricular tachycardia due to reentry of the ventricular impulse through the anomalous bundle of Kent.

During atrial fibrillation the ventricle is stimulated at a rapid rate via the accessory A-V bridge. Also, because the A-V junction is bypassed, the impulse does not experience the normal delay, and 1:1 conduction is seen with atrial flutter. These dangerously rapid ventricular rates may result in ventricular fibrillation.

A-V BYPASS—THE JAMES BUNDLE

Another accessory muscle bundle (the James bundle) accounts for some cases of accelerated A-V conduction with a normal QRS. This is an A-V

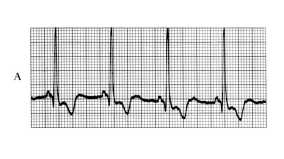

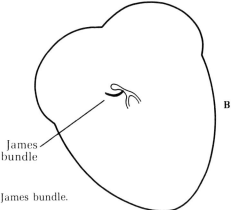

James
bundle

Fig. 12-6. A, Short P-R interval, normal QRS. **B,** James bundle.

nodal bypass extending from the atrium to the upper part of the His bundle. The pacemaker is the sinus node. Therefore the P waves are normal. However, the P-R interval is less than 0.12 second. Ventricular activation occurs normally via the bundle of His, and therefore the QRS complex will be of normal shape and duration. The extra A-V muscle bundle offers a nonrefractory retrograde pathway, so that these patients are subject to paroxysmal atrial tachycardia.

Abnormal intranodal A-V pathways may also possibly be present in patients who exhibit the ECG changes described.

The P-R interval in Fig. 12-6, *A,* is 0.08 second. The QRS duration is normal (0.10 second), and there is no delta wave. The normal delay at the A-V junction is not present. Therefore either a James bundle (Fig. 12-6, *B*) or an abnormal intranodal A-V pathway is present.

SUMMARY

Preexcitation is caused by atrioventricular muscular pathways other than the A-V junction. The ECG picture reflects early excitation of the ventricular muscle by a supraventricular impulse. In type A WPW syndrome the QRS is positive in V_1; in type B the QRS is negative in V_1.

The bundle of Kent (WPW syndrome) connects the left atrium with the left ventricle near the I-V septum (type A) or the right atrium with the right ventricle at the lateral border (type B). ECGs demonstrate the resultant short P-R interval and broadened QRS complex distorted by a delta wave.

The James bundle bypasses the A-V node (atrium to the bundle of His) and therefore a normal QRS complex with a short P-R interval will be observed.

These extra atrioventricular connections can cause supraventricular tachycardias due to reentry of the impulse across the anomalous bundle. This is possible because the extra muscle bundle becomes nonrefractory while the ventricle is still being activated.

TEST TRACINGS

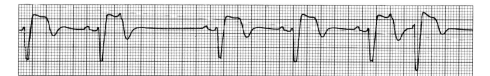

Fig. 12-7

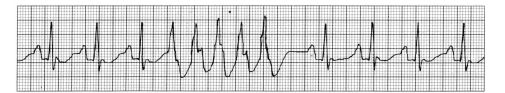

Fig. 12-8

Lead II

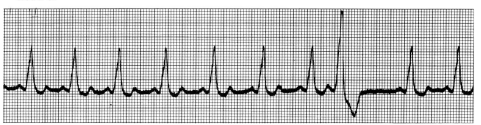

Fig. 12-9

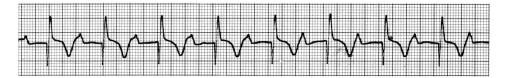

Fig. 12-10

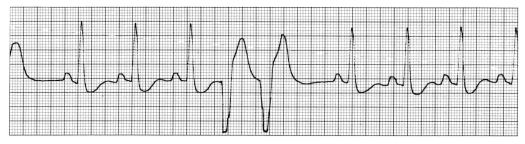

Fig. 12-11

ANSWERS

12-7   *PACs.* There are two P′ waves in this tracing. Both occur during the S-T segment, and the first P′ wave is not conducted.

12-8   *Paroxysmal ventricular tachycardia.* This burst of tachycardia begins with a PVC that remains in control of the ventricles for five beats. The sinus node then regains control.

12-9   *WPW syndrome.* The P-R interval in this tracing just borders on the normal. This, coupled with a broadened QRS complex and a delta wave, would indicate diagnosis of WPW syndrome. It is impossible to tell whether this is type A or type B without a full twelve-lead ECG.

12-10   *First-degree heart block.* The P-R interval is 0.32 to 0.36 second. All impulses are conducted but delayed across the A-V junction.

12-11   *Paired PVCs.* This is a more ominous sign than the single PVC.

13 Hypertrophies

A thickened muscle mass will have more cells than normal. There will therefore be more ions involved in the depolarization process (Fig. 13-1).

The depolarization process will take longer and the cardiac vector will become larger as the number of negative and positive ions increases. This is reflected in the ECG by a complex (atrial or ventricular) of longer duration and greater amplitude.

LEFT VENTRICULAR HYPERTROPHY

Normally the left ventricle is larger than the right, accounting for the small r and deep S waves in the right precordial leads and the small q and large R waves in the left precordial leads (Fig. 13-2).

When the left ventricle hypertrophies, the disproportion in size between the left and right ventricles is further increased and causes greater amplitude in the deflections, but a normal sequence of depolarization is retained.

ECG changes

1 *QRS amplitude:* The increase in the amplitude of the main ventricular vector is best reflected in the precordial leads. In leads facing the hypertrophied ventricle (V_6) a tall R wave (17 mm. or more) will usually be present. In leads facing the negative side of the activation (V_1) a deep S wave will be seen. The R wave in V_5 or V_6 plus the S wave in V_1 or V_2 will often be in excess of 40 mm.

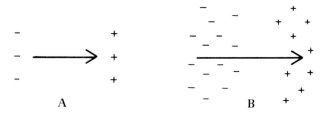

Fig. 13-1. A, Few cells and a small vector. **B,** Many cells and a large vector.

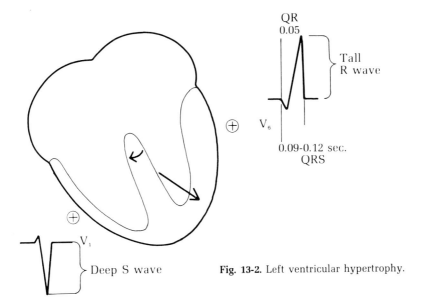

Fig. 13-2. Left ventricular hypertrophy.

2 *QRS duration:* The QRS interval lasts as long as the depolarization wave spreads through the ventricles (0.09 second or more). Prolongation of the QRS therefore represents delayed conduction of the impulse through the ventricles. In the presence of left ventricular hypertrophy, delay is due to the presence of more ventricular muscle tissue. A longer time is necessary for the current to completely depolarize the thickened muscle.

3 *Ventricular activation time (VAT):* In the thickened left ventricle a longer time is required for the current to reach the epicardium. Therefore in leads facing the left ventricle (V₆) the peak of the R wave is delayed (0.05 seconds or more), as shown in Fig. 13-2.

4 *T waves:* These may be of opposite polarity to that of the main QRS deflection. The repolarization process is changed because of delayed conduction through the ventricles.

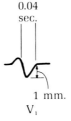

Fig. 13-3. Abnormal P wave in association with left ventricular hypertrophy.

5 *S-T segment displacement:* This displacement is in a direction opposite to that of the main QRS deflection.

6 *Left atrial involvement:* This may be associated with left ventricular hypertrophy and would be reflected in V_1 as a P wave with a terminal negative deflection of 1 mm. or more and a duration of 0.04 second or more (Fig. 13-3).

7 *Left axis deviation:* A deviation of -30 degrees or more may be present.

RIGHT VENTRICULAR HYPERTROPHY

Normally the electrical forces of the thick left ventricle dominate the ECG. When the right ventricle hypertrophies, this vectorial supremacy shifts. Therefore leads facing the right ventricle (V_1 and V_2) will resemble left ventricular leads. Conversely, the left ventricular leads (V_5 and V_6) will reflect ECG patterns that are ordinarily seen in right ventricular leads (Fig. 13-4).

ECG changes

1 *Precordial leads:* The configuration of the precordial leads is reversed, so that those facing the right ventricle will have tall R waves. Leads facing the left ventricle will have small r and deep S waves that reflect the dominance of the hypertrophied right ventricle.

2 *QRS duration:* The interval does not increase in duration. Even though the right ventricular wall is hypertrophied, it rarely exceeds the normal thickness of the left ventricular wall. Therefore the depolarization process will not take longer. Both ventricles will have completed the depolarization process at approximately the same time.

3 *Ventricular activation time (VAT):* The VAT occurs 0.04 second or more later in V_1 than in V_6 since the R wave peaks are reversed from the normal.

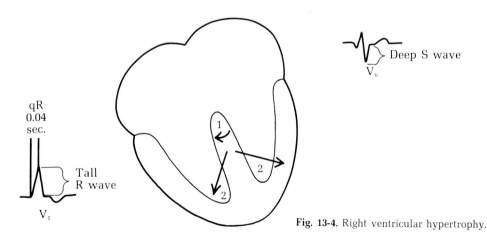

Fig. 13-4. Right ventricular hypertrophy.

4 *T wave:* The T wave is of opposite polarity to the main QRS deflection. This usually occurs when there is a change in the depolarization forces.

5 *Right atrial involvement:* This may be associated with right ventricular hypertrophy and would be reflected as tall, peaked P waves in leads II and III.

6 *Right axis deviation:* A deviation of +90 degrees or more is often present.

ATRIAL HYPERTROPHY

Normal atrial size will be reflected in the ECG by a P wave with a duration of not over 0.10 second and a height of 2.5 mm. or less. If either atrium is enlarged, these values will increase.

Left atrial hypertrophy

Left atrial hypertrophy is often accompanied by right ventricular hypertrophy, particularly when it occurs secondary to mitral stenosis, one of the more common causes of left atrial enlargement (Fig. 13-5).

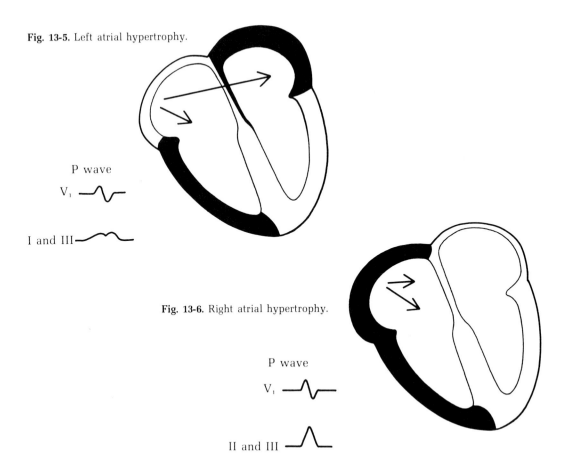

Fig. 13-5. Left atrial hypertrophy.

P wave

V₁

I and III

Fig. 13-6. Right atrial hypertrophy.

P wave

V₁

II and III

ECG changes

1 *Leads I and II:* "P mitrale" (broad notched P wave—more than 0.11 second in duration)
2 *Lead V_1:* Diphasic P wave with a broad, terminal, negative deflection

Right atrial hypertrophy

Right atrial hypertrophy is often due to chronic pulmonary disease and is frequently accompanied by a hypertrophied right ventricle (Fig. 13-6).

ECG changes

1 *Leads II and III:* Tall, peaked P wave more than 2.5 mm. in height
2 *Lead V_1:* Diphasic P wave, tall and peaked

TEST TRACINGS

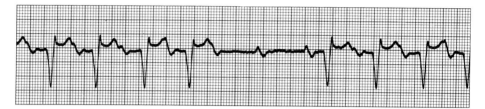

Fig. 13-7

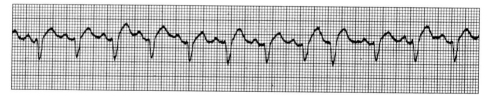

Fig. 13-8

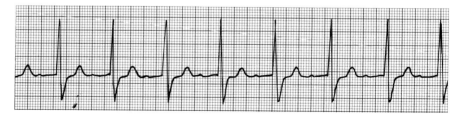

Fig. 13-9

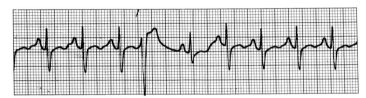

Fig. 13-10

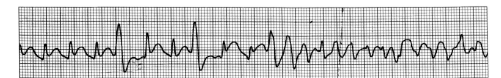

Fig. 13-11

ANSWERS

13-7 *Mobitz type II and left atrial hypertrophy.* The nonconducted P waves give us the opportunity to see the P-R interval of a conducted beat and the shape of the P wave. This is a second-degree A-V block (Mobitz type II) because some of the P waves are not conducted. The P-R interval of the conducted beat is 0.28 second. The QRS interval is also prolonged (0.16 second), indicating that the lesion is at or just below the bifurcation of the bundle of His. The duration of the P wave is 0.16 second. The wave is diphasic with a broad terminal negative deflection, indicative of left atrial hypertrophy.

13-8 *Sinus tachycardia with PACs.* The pause following the early ventricular complexes is not fully compensatory, indicating an atrial stimulus. The PAC causes the T wave to be taller and more peaked.

13-9 *First-degree A-V heart block.* Both the P-R interval and the QRS interval are prolonged, indicating that the lesion involves the bundle branches.

13-10 *Sinus tachycardia. PVC followed by postextrasystolic aberrancy.* The sinus rate is 112. There are QRS and T wave changes in the complex following the PVC due to the change in action potential caused by the shortening of the cycle length.

13-11 *Frequent PVCs resulting in ventricular fibrillation.* At a rate of 160 the underlying rhythm is either a sinus or an atrial tachycardia. There are PVCs occurring very early in diastole. When they are finally paired the result is ventricular fibrillation.

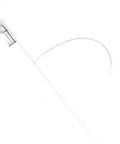

14 Dual rhythms

PARASYSTOLE

Parasystole is an arrhythmia in which two pacemakers are in command of the heart. One is the sinus node and the other is an ectopic center. This ectopic (parasystolic) focus continues its regular depolarization undisturbed by the sinus impulse.

In order for this parasystolic ventricular center to discharge regularly and escape being discharged by the sinus impulse, it must be "protected" from incoming stimuli (entrance block).

Entrance and exit block

One of the effects of ischemia on the myocardial cells is the reduction of the resting membrane potential and the creation of areas of decremental conduction.

Reduction of the resting membrane potential lowers the rate of rise and amplitude of the action potential. The amplitude of the action potential determines the conduction velocity. Therefore it is possible that a group of cells in the His-Purkinje system that have lost their normal resting mem-

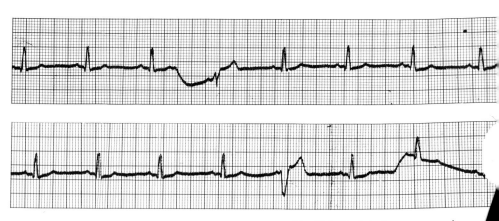

Fig. 14-1. Ventricular parasystole

brane potential are able to spread weak but effective depolarization currents to adjacent cells (decremental conduction) but are unable to be depolarized from an external stimulus (entrance block). The current may also be too weak to be conducted to neighboring cells (exit block).

ECG changes

1. The ectopic complexes are not accurately coupled to the sinus beats. That is, they are independent of the sinus mechanism and do not require preceding activity for their initiation.
2. Fusion beats sometimes occur, indicating independent ectopic activity.
3. Since the rhythm of the ectopic focus is regular, the time interval between the parasystolic complexes will be constant. The ectopic focus will depolarize regularly but may not manifest a complex each time due to refractory ventricular tissue. Therefore the longest ectopic interval should be divisible by the shortest ectopic interval, indicating a regular rhythm.

The coupling intervals of the PVCs in Fig. 14-1 are different in each case. The shortest interval between ectopic beats (the last two) may be evenly divided into the longest interval, indicating that the ectopic focus is undisturbed by the sinus-conducted ventricular impulses. The absence of fixed coupling indicates that the ventricular ectopic beat is not due to reentry. That is, it is in no way dependent upon a sinus-conducted impulse for its occurrence. The first and last ectopic beats are fusion beats, further confirming the independence of the ectopic focus.

A-V DISSOCIATION

In A-V dissociation there are two pacemakers, one for the atria (usually the sinus node) and one for the ventricles (usually the A-V node). The rates of these two pacemakers are slightly different, the nodal pacemaker usually being somewhat faster (Fig. 14-2).

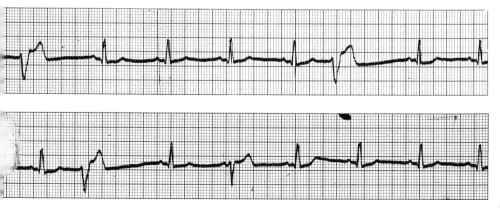

(continuous strips).

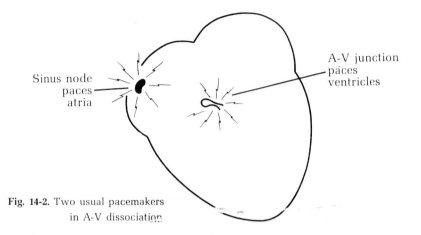

Fig. 14-2. Two usual pacemakers
in A-V dissociation

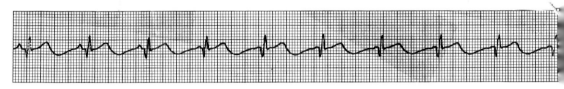

Fig. 14-3. A-V dissociation

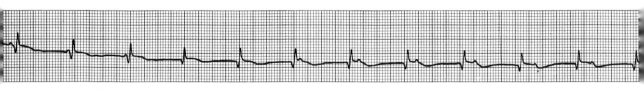

Fig. 14-4. A-V dissociation

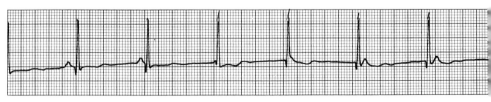

Fig. 14-5. A-V dissociation

The term "A-V dissociation" does not apply to a pathological block of the A-V node as seen in complete heart block but rather to a usurpation of ventricular control by an irritable A-V node (an active rhythm) or to the relinquishment of control by a slow sinus node (a passive rhythm).

The sinus node will occasionally control the ventricles if it finds the A-V nodal tissue nonrefractory. When the P wave occurs far enough beyond the QRS complex to control the next ventricular beat, it effects what is called *ventricular capture*. The capture beat may be of a slightly different shape from the nodal beat.

A-V dissociation as an active rhythm

In the tracing shown in Fig. 14-3 the A-V node has taken over actively at a rate of 70. The atrial rate remains at 67. There is A-V dissociation until the A-V node slows down again and allows the sinus node to dominate. The P waves disappear into the QRS, but they never emerge on the other side. This occurs because the two rates are so similar, and the A-V node slows down before the P wave can overtake the QRS complex.

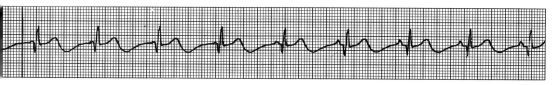

(continuous strips).

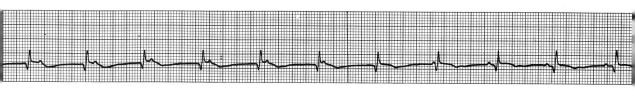

(continuous strips).

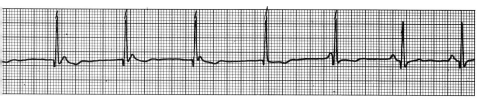

(continuous strips).

At the time A-V dissociation begins in Fig. 14-4, the sinus node has a rate of 70 and the A-V node has a rate of 74, so that this is another active rhythm. The P wave "walks through" the QRS complex and emerges on the other side. The sinus node then speeds up slightly, causing the P wave to drop back into the QRS, emerge on the proper side, and again regain control of the ventricle (ventricular capture).

A-V dissociation as a passive rhythm

In passive A-V dissociation the A-V node paces the heart because the sinus node has either failed or is too slow. In Fig. 14-5 the sinus node slows slightly from a rate of 58 to 55. The A-V node then assumes control at its own rate of 58. The P waves begin to get closer and closer to the QRS, enter it, and emerge on the other side. The two nodes then beat at approximately the same rate, and the sinus node regains control again only after it has accelerated to a rate of 67.

TEST TRACINGS

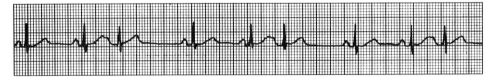

Fig. 14-6

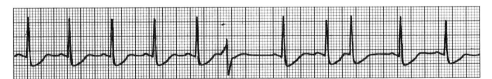

Fig. 14-7

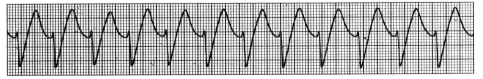

Fig. 14-8

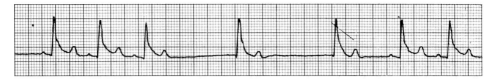

Fig. 14-9

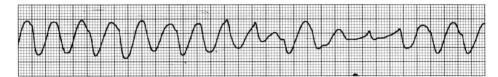

Fig. 14-10

ANSWERS

14-6 *Trigeminal PACs.* There is a PAC after each pair of normal sinus beats. The P′ wave distorts the preceding T wave. The P′-R interval is long (0.22 second) because the ectopic stimulus occurs during the relative refractory period, causing a delay in conduction through the A-V junction.

14-7 *PVC and a premature junctional contraction.* The PVC is easily identified because of its broad, different shape and its full compensatory pause. The next premature complex is of the same shape as the sinus-conducted complexes. Therefore the focus must be above the bifurcation of the bundle of His. There is not a full compensatory pause; therefore the sinus node must have been activated early by the ectopic focus. Since an ectopic P′ wave is not visible, it must be hidden in the QRS.

14-8 *Ventricular tachycardia.* The ventricular rate is 110. There are no P waves visible, and there are no ventricular fusion beats. This could therefore also be a supraventricular tachycardia with aberrant ventricular conduction.

14-9 *Atrial standstill with junctional escape.* There is a sinus exit block resulting in atrial standstill. After a pause the A-V junction begins to pace the heart (junctional escape). There are no P waves evident during this time (atrial standstill). After two junctional escape beats the sinus node resumes its role as pacemaker.

14-10 *Ventricular fibrillation.* The onset of this tracing might be termed ventricular flutter since there is some repetition of the wide, bizarre complexes. Complete electrical chaos soon is evident.

15 Fusion beats

In electrocardiography the term "fusion" is used to indicate that two vectors from two different foci that have started to move at almost the same time have met within the muscle mass of either the atrium (atrial fusion) or the ventricle (ventricular fusion). Contrary to what is sometimes thought, the term "fusion beat" does not mean that a P wave has occurred during the QRS complex.

Electrophysiology

The terms "atrial fusion" or "ventricular fusion" imply that there are two vectors or currents active simultaneously within the atria or ventricles. These two vectors simply cancel each other out, causing a complex of lower amplitude. Fig. 15-1 shows that when the depolarization process is initiated from two different sites within the atria or the ventricles, opposing cell masses become immediately negative, thus making it impossible for a large number of negative ions to oppose a large number of positive ions. There-

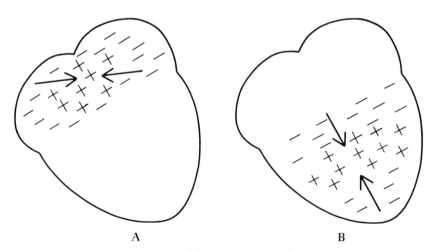

Fig. 15-1. A, Atrial fusion. B, Ventricular fusion.

fore the vector can never at any moment in the process be very big, since it is the number of negative cells opposing positive cells that determines the strength of the vector.

Atrial fusion beats occur most frequently when an ectopic atrial focus and the sinus node discharge simultaneously or almost simultaneously (Fig. 15-1, *A*). Ventricular fusion beats most often occur when an ectopic ventricular focus discharges at or almost at the same time as normal conduction begins at the A-V junction (Fig. 15-1, *B*).

ECG changes

1 *Complexes of low amplitude:* Complexes of low amplitude are caused by two smaller vectors canceling each other out.
2 *Complexes of shorter duration:* Complexes of shorter duration are seen in both P fusion and in QRS fusion beats. Two electrical forces cause the depolarization process to be completed more quickly.

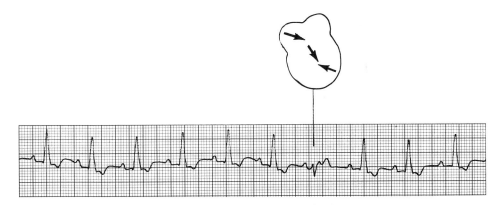

Fig. 15-2. Ventricular fusion.

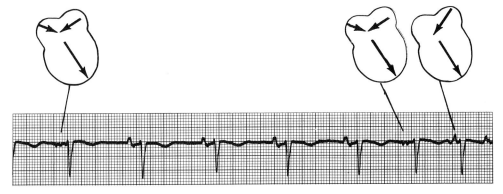

Fig. 15-3. Atrial fusion.

VENTRICULAR FUSION

In the tracing shown in Fig. 15-2 an end-diastolic PVC is not early enough to completely capture the ventricle. The ectopic vector begins to activate the ventricle at almost the same time that the normal vector has begun its course down the I-V septum. The electrical forces thus cancel each other out, and a complex of lesser amplitude is produced. The duration of the depolarization process has been shortened from 0.12 to 0.05 second. Notice also that the aberrant ventricular activity has caused an aberrant T wave.

ATRIAL FUSION

The first two PACs in the tracing shown in Fig. 15-3 are not early enough to escape a collision with the normal sinus impulse. The decreased amplitude is recorded as a line that is almost isoelectric, except for two slight negative deflections. The last atrial complex on the tracing is a PAC that precedes the sinus impulse and is thus early enough to command the atria.

TEST TRACINGS

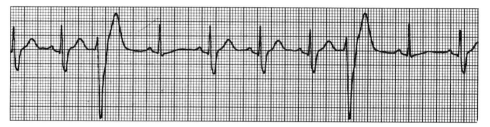

Fig. 15-4

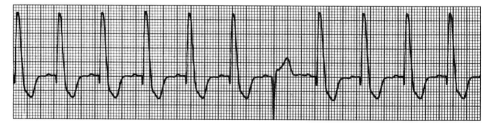

Fig. 15-5

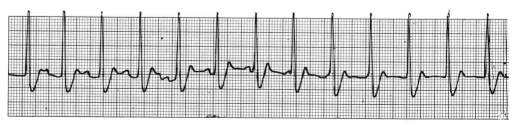

Fig. 15-6

ANSWERS

15-4 *PVCs in association with intermittent bundle branch block.* The ventricular complex following the PVC is normal in contour and duration as opposed to the other sinus-conducted beats with their broad terminal S waves. Evidently the ventricular ectopic stimulus does not activate the A-V junction, giving it time to rest and conduct the next stimulus normally.

15-5 *Ventricular fusion.* The P-R interval of the narrow complex is slightly less than the dominant P-R interval, indicating that an ectopic focus discharged in the ventricle just before the normal sinus stimulus reached the I-V septum. The two vectors may meet, causing a complex of lesser amplitude and duration, or the ectopic focus may be of septal origin and may dominate the ventricles completely.

15-6 *A-V dissociation.* The A-V nodal rate is 110. Therefore this is an active rhythm. The rate of the sinus node is 100. The P waves can be seen to get closer and closer to the QRS, disappear into the QRS, and emerge on the other side to begin overtaking the QRS again. The negative ventricular complex may represent ventricular capture rather than an ectopic beat. Sometimes the capture beats are shaped differently from the nodal rhythm. The fact that this negative complex is barely 0.08 second in duration would suggest capture.

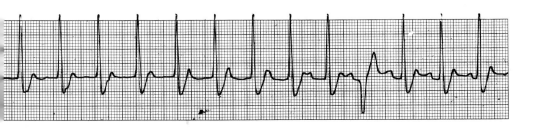

16 Pacemakers

Normally the sinus node paces the heart with a regular, rhythmic impulse. This impulse passes into the ventricles via the A-V node, bundle of His, and right and left bundle branches. There is normally a slight delay of approximately 0.11 second in impulse transmission at the A-V node. This delay allows for the atrial contents to empty into the ventricles before they contract.

Some disturbances of normal heart rate, rhythm, or conduction may be corrected with an electronic pacemaker. For example, the sinus node may fail or the A-V node may be pathologically blocked, preventing impulses from entering the ventricles. The heart can then be paced artificially, and the rate and strength of the stimulus can be controlled.

TYPES OF PACEMAKERS
Fixed-rate pacemaker

A fixed-rate (continuous asynchronous) pacemaker fires at a set rate regardless of the patient's own intrinsic rhythm. There is the danger that a pacemaker stimulus may fall within the relative refractory or vulnerable period, causing a serious ventricular arrhythmia (Fig. 16-1).

Demand pacemaker

The demand pacemaker fires only if the patient's own rate falls below a preset level. It functions by determining the R-R interval on the ECG. This interval is evaluated electronically, and if it is found to be too long, the pacemaker escapes.

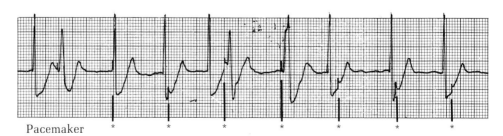

Pacemaker

Fig. 16-1. Fixed-rate pacemaker in competition with the patient's own rhythm.

There are two types of demand pacemakers, the QRS inhibited and the QRS triggered. The QRS-inhibited pacemaker (Fig. 16-2) will not fire when sensing an R wave. The QRS-triggered pacemaker (Fig. 16-3) senses the R wave and fires in the refractory period of the ventricular complex. The pre-set firing time is measured from this stimulus. If an R wave does not occur before the preset time, the pacemaker escapes and stimulates the ventricles.

Refractory period of the demand pacemaker

An artificial refractory period is a feature of all demand pacemakers. This refractory period is the time during which the pacemaker electrode does not sense a stimulus. It should be shorter than the shortest possible coupling interval, for if it fails to sense a very premature extrasystole, it may generate a stimulus that could fall on the T wave of that extrasystole. The pacemaker refractory time is usually about 0.4 second.

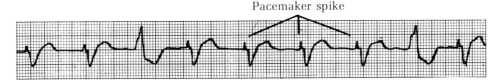

Pacemaker spike

Fig. 16-2. QRS-inhibited pacemaker.

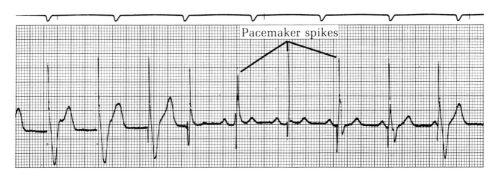

Pacemaker spikes

Fig. 16-3. QRS-triggered pacemaker.

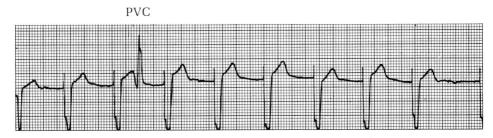

PVC

Fig. 16-4. Premature ventricular contraction occurring within the pacemaker refractory period.

In Fig. 16-4 the PVC falls within the refractory period of the pacemaker, that is, within the first 0.4 second after the pacemaker spike. The PVC is therefore not sensed by the pacemaker, which continues uninterrupted at a rate of 82.

Synchronized pacemaker

The synchronized pacemaker is the most physiological of the pacemakers. It is synchronous with the patient's P wave. There is an electrode in the atrium as well as in the ventricle. The atrial electrode is a sensor that detects the atrial depolarization and passes this information on to the ventricular electrode, which discharges after a slight delay. The delay allows the atria to empty their contents into the ventricles, creating an approximation of normal synchronous cardiac function.

PACEMAKER SPIKES

The spike from a bipolar pacemaker is small (Fig. 16-5). The spike from a unipolar pacemaker is large (Fig. 16-6).

METHODS OF INSERTION

The pacemaker electrode can be placed in contact with the myocardium by the transvenous, transthoracic, or epicardial method.

Transvenous method

A transvenous pacemaker may be temporary or permanent. A bipolar electrode catheter is placed in the apex of the right ventricle in close contact with the endocardial surface. The catheter is inserted under fluoroscopic control. A cutdown technique is used. The pacing catheter that is threaded into the right ventricle may be introduced via the jugular, basilic, femoral, or cephalic vein (Fig. 16-7). The temporary transvenous pacemaker is attached to an external battery unit, and the control battery of the permanent transvenous pacemaker is inserted surgically into the subcutaneous tissue of the chest.

Most transvenous pacemakers are placed within the right ventricular cavity. However, the pacemaker catheter may be placed in the atrium in the absence of a pathological process in the A-V node. The electrical events of the ventricles would then occur normally, synchronized with the atrial contraction. Cardiac output would be improved by this method, but the catheter position is somewhat less reliable.

Transthoracic method

A large needle is used to insert the electrodes directly into the ventricle through the chest wall. This is an emergency procedure and is preferred to the external pacemaker.

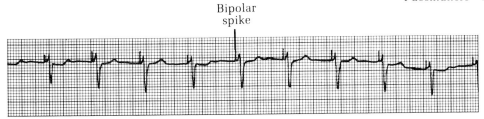

Fig. 16-5. Bipolar pacemaker spike.

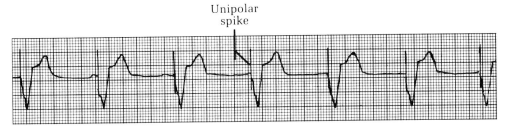

Fig. 16-6. Unipolar pacemaker spike.

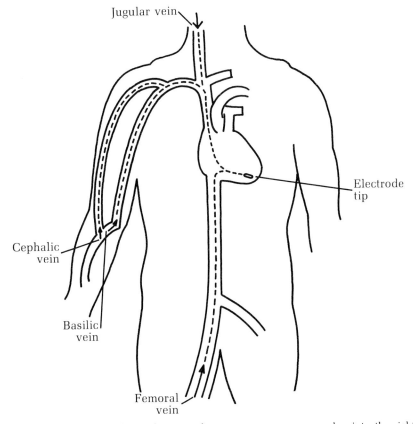

Fig. 16-7. Routes commonly used to introduce a transvenous pacemaker into the right ventricle.

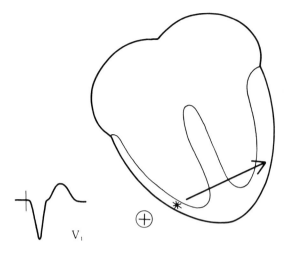

Fig. 16-8. Ventricular complex with the pacemaker electrode in the right ventricle.

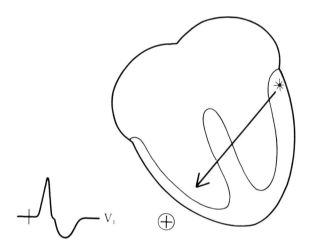

Fig. 16-9. Ventricular complex with the pacemaker electrode in the left ventricle.

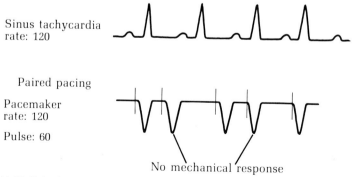

Fig. 16-10. Paired pacing.

Epicardial method

A thoracotomy is necessary for this procedure, in which electrodes are sutured to the epicardium. The pulse generator is buried in a subcutaneous pocket. The pacing mode may be either synchronous or nonsynchronous.

VENTRICULAR COMPLEXES PRODUCED BY THE PACEMAKER SPIKE

If the tip of the pacemaker catheter lies in the apex of the right ventricle, a left bundle branch pattern will result (Fig. 16-8).

If the pacemaker electrode is implanted in the left ventricle, a right bundle branch pattern will result (Fig. 16-9).

INDICATIONS FOR A PACEMAKER
Myocardial infarction

Temporary pacing has become the treatment of choice for patients with transient heart block or refractory sinus slowing that is associated with myocardial infarction.

Stokes-Adams syndrome

Permanent pacing is favored for patients with complete heart block and Stokes-Adams attacks.

Ectopic beats

Temporary pacing is being used successfully in the treatment of ectopic arrhythmias. The heart is paced at a rate exceeding the spontaneous heart rate in an effort to suppress the ectopic pacemaker. This is known as "overdrive suppression."

PAIRED PACING

Since 1885 it has been known that a PVC following closely upon a normal beat does not result in a mechanical contraction. However, the beat following this ineffective depolarization has a greater force of contraction. This is because of the longer filling time allowed by the combination of a full compensatory pause and a mechanically ineffective extrasystole.

Paired pacing is one of the less common ways of decreasing the effective rate of arrhythmias. In this technique, two electrical stimuli are delivered to the heart at short, predetermined intervals. The first stimulus causes depolarization followed by a ventricular contraction. During the repolarization process there is a 50 millisecond (msec.) period during the T wave in which an electrical stimulus would provoke a QRS response but not a mechanical contraction. The second stimulus is therefore set to fall in this phase of repolarization, thus resulting in an electrical but not a mechanical event (Fig. 16-10).

This technique carries with it special hazards in the presence of myocardial infarction, particularly because of the lowered fibrillatory threshold.

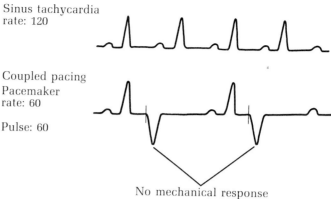

Sinus tachycardia
rate: 120

Coupled pacing
Pacemaker
rate: 60

Pulse: 60

No mechanical response

Fig. 16-11. Coupled pacing.

COUPLED PACING

Coupled pacing makes use of the patient's own sinus rhythm. A ventricular bigeminy is produced by introducing an electrical stimulus closely coupled to the patient's beat. This results in an increased stroke volume due to a full compensatory pause and a long diastolic filling time. The heart rate is reduced by half since the electrically stimulated PVC is of negligible magnitude due to insufficient recovery of the ventricular muscle and insignificant ventricular filling (Fig. 16-11).

PACEMAKER MALFUNCTION

In order for the pacemaker electrode to effectively deliver its stimulus to the myocardium, there are certain conditions that must be fulfilled:

1 The electrode must be in contact with the myocardium.
2 The pulse generator must be functioning properly.
3 The electrode must be intact.
4 The threshold potential of the myocardial cells must not be greater than the amplitude delivered by the pacemaker.

If any one of the above conditions is not fulfilled, pacemaker malfunction will result.

The pacemaker blip in Fig. 16-12 is the very tall spike occurring regularly through the strip. Although this is a demand pacemaker, it is firing irrespective of the patient's inherent rate. This is a dangerous situation since it fires during the T wave or vulnerable period.

Fig. 16-13 depicts another example of pacemaker malfunction. The pacemaker is set to fire if the patient's rate falls below 68. In the center portion of this tracing the patient's ventricular rate is 72, but the pacemaker is discharging nonetheless. The pacemaker blip can be seen on the T wave. Finally, there is capture, and the pacemaker is in command at a rate slower than the patient's.

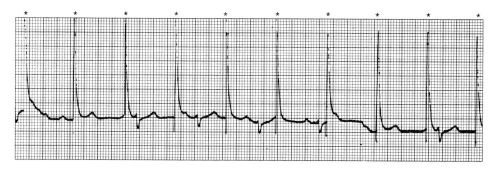

Fig. 16-12. Pacemaker malfunction.

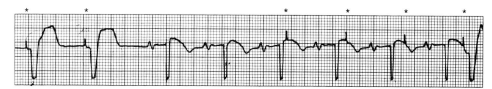

Fig. 16-13. Pacemaker malfunction.

Checking for battery failure

The pulse generators of most permanent pacemakers have a battery life of approximately 30 months, but many physicians routinely replace the pulse generator after 20 months because a significant percentage fail early.

Evaluation of a permanent demand pacemaker often requires that the pacemaker be temporarily converted to a fixed-rate modality, particularly when the intrinsic rate is faster than the preset pacemaker rate. This is accomplished by placing a magnet on the skin overlying the pulse generator. Most units have been designed so that the demand mode may be suppressed or disengaged by the use of a magnet.

TEST TRACINGS

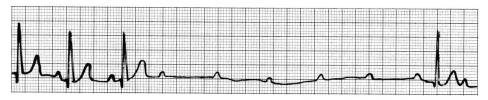

Fig. 16-14

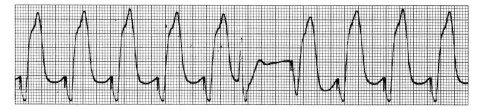

Fig. 16-15

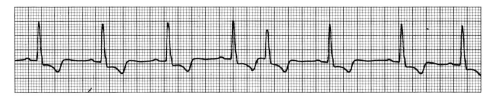

Fig. 16-16

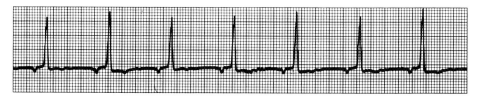

Fig. 16-17

ANSWERS

16-14 *Sudden complete heart block with junctional escape.* A-V conduction abruptly fails in this tracing. The complexes at the beginning of the strip are conducted with a P-R interval of 0.16 second. There is a long period with no ventricular activity and then junctional escape. This patient has Stokes-Adams syndrome and was a candidate for a pacemaker.

16-15 *Demand pacemaker.* The pacemaker spike can be seen just before the ventricular complex. There is a PVC that is sensed by the pacemaker, and thus there is a delay in the next firing.

16-16 *PAC.* The PAC in this tracing is not immediately apparent. The premature ventricular complex is not followed by a full compensatory pause. This causes one to search for a PAC. If the T waves are closely examined and their shapes compared, the inverted T wave preceding the premature complex will appear to be more peaked. A P' wave occurs in the T wave.

16-17 *Coronary sinus rhythm.* In lead II a negative P wave indicates that the pacemaker is in the vicinity of the A-V node or in the bundle of His. Since the P'-R interval is normal (0.14 second), the impulse must have experienced the normal delay at the A-V junction. The focus is therefore above the A-V node, possibly in the coronary sinus on the floor of the right atrium.

17 Myocardial infarction

The results of an occlusion of a coronary artery will depend upon the state of the collateral circulation and the location of the occlusion. Cellular changes begin immediately. Unless blood flow is reestablished to the ischemic tissue, more and more cells will succumb to the effects of anoxia. Approximately 20 minutes after the occlusion, the first necrotic cells appear. Until this point, recovery would have been rapid with a reestablished blood flow, but necrosis is irreversible.

These irreversibly injured necrotic cells lie toward the center of the infarct. Surrounding this center is an area of tissue that is nonfunctional or unable to repolarize due to metabolic and ionic changes. Ischemic, though functioning, tissue is closest to the normally perfused areas at the periphery.

These histological changes in the myocardium are reflected in the ECG tracing shown in Fig. 17-1.

ISCHEMIA

Ischemia of tissue surrounding the infarct causes a reversal of the T wave. Because the depolarization process is changed due to local ischemia, the repolarization process is also altered.

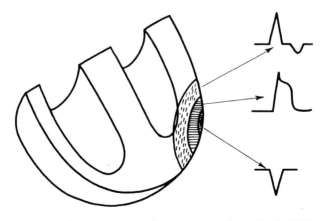

Fig. 17-1. Ischemia, injury, and necrosis as reflected in the ECG.

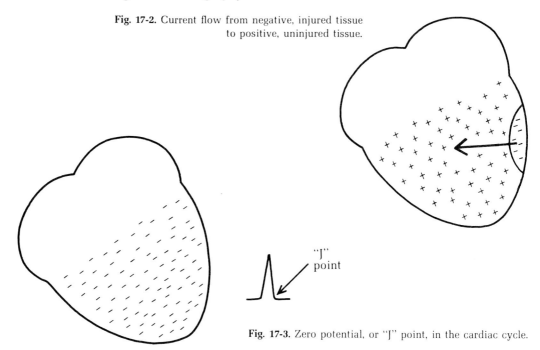

Fig. 17-2. Current flow from negative, injured tissue to positive, uninjured tissue.

Fig. 17-3. Zero potential, or "J" point, in the cardiac cycle.

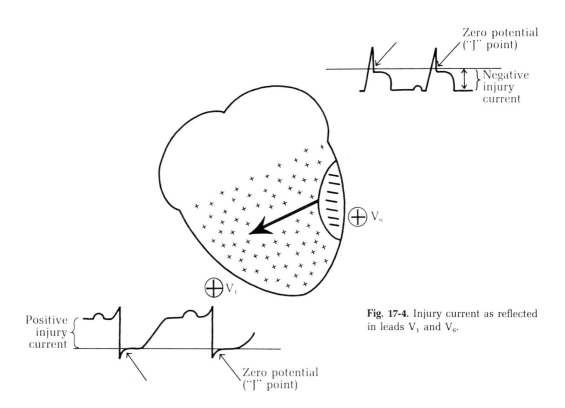

Fig. 17-4. Injury current as reflected in leads V_1 and V_6.

INJURY

Because of severe ischemia and lack of nutrients, the tissue immediately surrounding the center of the infarct is nonfunctional. It receives its blood supply from the collateral circulation. This is sufficient to keep it alive but insufficient to maintain membrane integrity.

Healthy cardiac cells will remain polarized until a stimulus triggers them to depolarize.

Nonfunctional or injured cardiac cells will begin to repolarize with the rest of the heart. However, a loss of membrane integrity makes it impossible for them to hold their charges. These charges, or ions, will then leak away from the cell. This exodus of ions from the injured tissue is called a *current of injury* (Fig. 17-2).

The completion of the QRS complex represents the zero potential, or "J" point, since at this time all cells (including those that are injured) are depolarized, and no current is flowing. To determine the zero potential line of the ECG, a horizontal line is drawn through the J points (Fig. 17-3).

When repolarization commences (the T wave), the injury current begins to flow, causing a displacement of the T-P segment. In other words the J point and the S-T segment will not be on the same line as the T-P segment. Leads closest to the infarct will sense a current flowing away from the positive electrode (a negative injury current). The T-P segment is thus displaced downward, since it is this segment that is affected by the abnormal current. This causes the S-T segment to appear to be elevated (Fig. 17-4).

Leads on the opposite side of the heart will sense a current flowing toward the positive electrode (a positive injury current). The T-P segment is thus displaced upward, causing the S-T segment to appear to be depressed (Fig. 17-4).

Leads on the opposite side of the heart will sense a current flowing toward the positive electrode (a positive injury current). This will be reflected in the ECG as a depressed S-T segment, as seen in Fig. 17-4.

NECROSIS

Necrotic tissue has no polarity. This area of the infarct therefore acts as a window through which the electrode "sees" a current moving away from the infarcted area. This abnormally directed QRS vector causes a Q wave with a duration of more than 0.04 second in leads facing the infarcted area (Fig. 17-5).

*   *   *

Myocardial necrosis, injury, and ischemia (Fig. 17-6) may be present at the same time, and the ECG manifestations of all three states may occur simultaneously (Fig. 17-7). The positive electrode closest to the infarcted area will reflect the infarction most prominently.

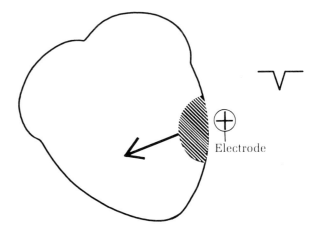

Fig. 17-5. Q wave is seen best in leads directly over the necrotic tissue.

A

B

Fig. 17-6. A, Ischemia. **B,** Injury. **C,** Death.

C

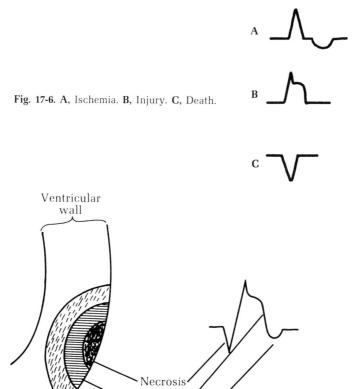

Fig. 17-7. All three grades of injury may be seen in one lead.

ANTERIOR WALL INFARCTION

The anterior wall is divided into four sections: anterobasal, anterolateral, anteroseptal, and apical. Infarctions can occur in all four areas.

Anterobasal infarct

The anterobasal or hi-lateral infarct is best seen in leads I and aV_L and is due to an occlusion of a branch of the circumflex artery (Fig. 17-8).

Anterolateral infarct

The anterolateral infarct is best seen in the precordial leads overlying the infarct (V_4, V_5, and V_6). It is caused by an occlusion of the diagonal branch of the left anterior descending branch of the left coronary artery (Fig. 17-9).

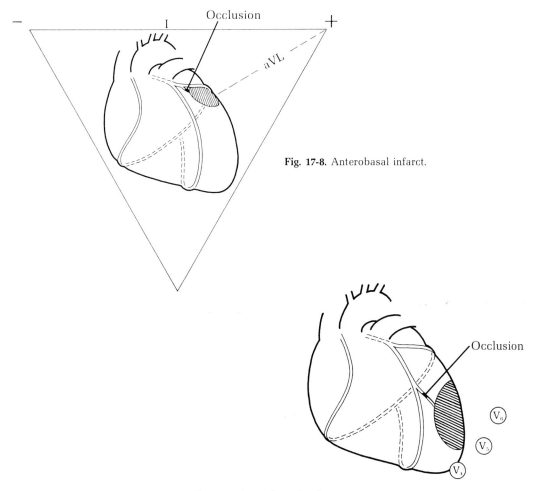

Fig. 17-8. Anterobasal infarct.

Fig. 17-9. Anterolateral infarct.

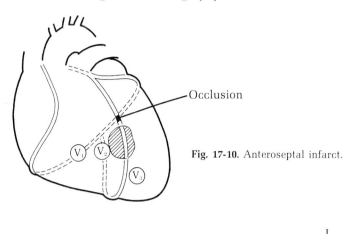

Fig. **17-10.** Anteroseptal infarct.

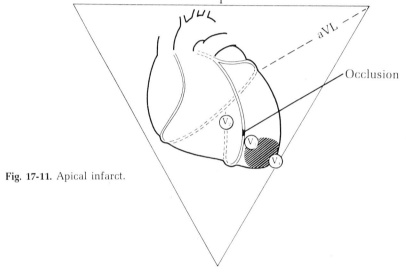

Fig. **17-11.** Apical infarct.

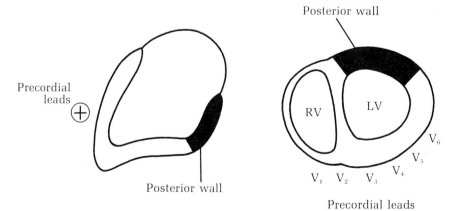

Fig. **17-12.** Posterior wall infarction.

Anteroseptal infarct

The anteroseptal or anterior infarct is best seen in leads V_1, V_2, and V_3 and is due to an occlusion of the left anterior descending branch of the left coronary artery (Fig. 17-10).

Apical infarct

The apical infarct is best seen in leads I and aV_L and in the precordial leads V_2, V_3, and V_4. It is caused by an occlusion of the left anterior descending branch of the left coronary artery (Fig. 17-11).

POSTERIOR WALL INFARCTION

Posterior wall infarction is caused by an occlusion of either the right coronary artery or a branch of the circumflex artery.

The precordial leads will show reciprocal changes due to loss of posterior forces. Therefore, instead of an abnormal Q wave, there will be a tall, broad initial R. Instead of an S-T segment elevation due to an injury current traveling away from the electrode, there will be an S-T segment depression due to an injury current traveling toward the electrode. The T wave will be upright rather than inverted (Fig. 17-12).

DIAPHRAGMATIC INFARCTION

The diaphragmatic infarction is best seen in the limb leads II, III, and aV_F. These are the leads in which the positive electrode "faces up" toward the infarcted area (Fig. 17-13). It is caused by an occlusion of the right coronary artery.

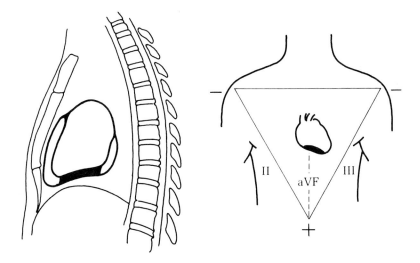

Fig. 17-13. Diaphragmatic infarction.

LATERAL WALL INFARCTION

Lateral wall infarction is caused by an occlusion of the circumflex artery or branch of the left anterior descending artery. The lateral wall of the heart faces up toward the left shoulder. Therefore the positive electrodes that face this side of the heart will detect the infarction best. These leads are I, aV_L, V_5, and V_6 (Fig. 17-14).

STAGES OF RECOVERY

During the acute phases of infarction, when there is a greater amount of nonfunctional and necrotic tissue, S-T segment displacements and QRS changes are seen. As the nonfunctional tissue either dies or becomes functional again, the S-T segment displacements disappear and are replaced by inverted T waves, an indication of secondary ischemia (the nonfunctional tissue in becoming functional will still be ischemic).

These processes take anywhere from several days to 3 weeks. As healing progresses, the Q wave regresses. In most cases it will persist permanently. However, in some cases when the dead tissue becomes fibrosed and turns to scar tissue, the area may be so small that it is not demonstrated on the ECG.

PERICARDITIS

Since deviation of the S-T segment and inversion of the T wave are also the features of myocardial infarction, we have included pericarditis in this chapter.

Anatomical aspects

The heart is enveloped in two membranes, the visceral and the parietal pericardium (Fig. 17-15). Inflammation of either one or both of these membranes is called pericarditis.

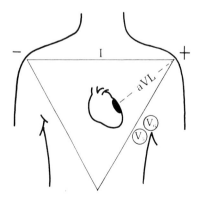

Fig. 17-14. Lateral wall infarction.

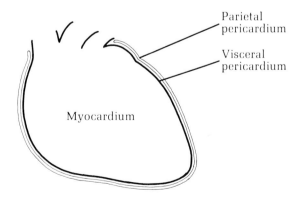

Fig. 17-15. Pericardium.

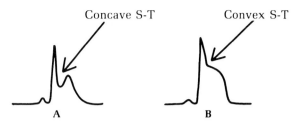

Fig. 17-16. A, Pericarditis. B, Myocardial infarction.

Electrophysiology

The epicardial surface beneath the inflamed area will be unable to polarize. There will therefore be an injury current (elevated S-T segment) in leads reflecting the involved area. As the disease becomes less acute, the upward displacement of the S-T segment disappears, returning to the isoelectric line or below it, and the T wave becomes inverted. The T wave changes occur during the subacute stage and are attributed to delayed repolarization of the epicardium, which is usually the first to repolarize.

ECG changes

1 *S-T segment:* In myocardial infarction there is, in most cases, reciprocal S-T segment depression. For example, if there is elevation of the S-T segment in a lead over the infarction, there will be a reciprocal depression of the S-T segment in a lead over the opposite surface of the heart. In acute pericarditis this reciprocal S-T depression rarely occurs. Rather, because of the diffuse nature of pericarditis, the S-T segment elevation will be seen in all leads reflecting epicardial potentials. The S-T segment also looks different in pericarditis, taking a concave form as opposed to the convex form seen in myocardial infarction (Fig. 17-16).

2 *T wave:* In pericarditis the T wave may be inverted in all three standard leads (I, II, and III). This is significant and seldom occurs in myocardial infarction. Usually in pericarditis the T wave inversion will occur in leads I and II.

3 *Q waves:* The characteristic Q waves of myocardial infarction do not occur in pericarditis.

TEST TRACINGS

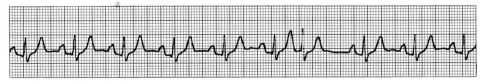

Fig. 17-17

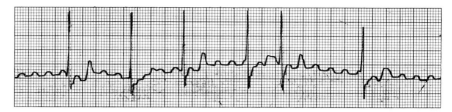

Fig. 17-18

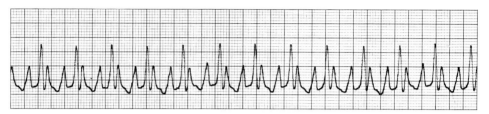

Fig. 17-19

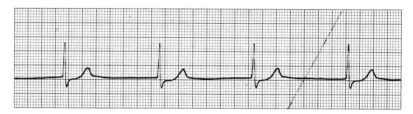

Fig. 17-20

ANSWERS

17-17 *PAC.* The PAC in this tracing occurs on a T wave, causing it to be taller and more peaked.

17-18 *Atrial flutter with variable block.* The atrial rate is 300. Although there is an isoelectric line between each P'-P' interval, this is diagnosed as atrial flutter because of the rapid atrial rate. Perhaps another lead would show the characteristic sawtooth pattern. The A-V block varies from 3:1 to 6:1.

17-19 *Atrial tachycardia with 2:1 A-V conduction.* The atrial rate is 220. The ventricular rate is 110. One of the P' waves is partially hidden in the QRS complex. Its downstroke can be seen emerging from the S wave. The P waves are excessively tall and broad, indicating atrial hypertrophy.

17-20 *Junctional bradycardia.* The rate is 43. There are no P waves visible since they are hidden in the QRS complex.

18 Drugs and electrolytes and their effect on the ECG

SYMPATHETIC NERVOUS SYSTEM

The sympathetic nerve (Fig. 18-1) is composed of a preganglionic fiber, where the hormone acetylcholine is released; a cholinergic receptor (receiver of acetylcholine); a postganglionic fiber, where the hormone norepinephrine is released; and an adrenergic receptor (receiver of norepinephrine; from the word "adrenal"). The adrenergic receptor is located on the effector cell. These adrenergic receptors have been divided into *alpha* receptors and *beta* receptors.

Sequence of action of the sympathetic nerve

An action potential or sympathomimetic drug releases norepinephrine from the nerve ending. The alpha and beta adrenergic receptors then trigger a series of responses that finally result in an acceleration of the rate of the sinus node or a contraction or relaxation of a smooth muscle.

Terminology

norepinephrine Mediator of the sympathetic nerve.
sympathomimetic drugs (mimetic = mimic) Mimic the effects of stimuli to the sympathetic nervous system by stimulating the nerve ending.

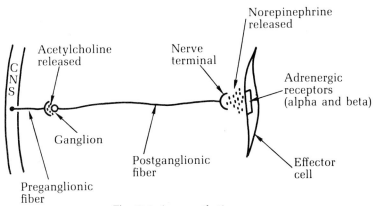

Fig. 18-1. A sympathetic nerve.

catecholamines A particular group of sympathetic endogenous mediators; dopamine, norepinephrine, and epinephrine are included in this category.

sympatholytic drugs (Gr. lytikos = dissolving) Block the effects of the sympathetic nervous system at the nerve terminal or at the receptor site (alpha or beta).

adrenergic Refers to the receptors (alpha and beta) for these drugs; here in the effector cell or end organ the hormone norepinephrine is received and the activation of muscular contraction is begun.

adrenergic drugs Act at this effector site.

alpha and beta receptors Specific receptive sites within the effector cell or end organ.

chronotropic effect Refers to heart rate and may be either positive or negative.

inotropic effect Refers to myocardial contractility and may be either positive or negative.

Adrenergic receptors and the cardiovascular system

The heart is subserved by beta receptors. The responses of the heart to adrenergic stimuli are as follows:

1 Increased rate of the sinus node and the rest of the conductive system (positive chronotropic effect)
2 Enhanced myocardial contractility (positive inotropic effect)
3 Increased metabolic activity

Arterial vasoconstriction is considered to be a function of the alpha receptors. *Arterial and venous dilatation* is a function of the beta receptors, and *venous constriction* is a function of both alpha and beta receptors. The vascular bed of the kidneys has primarily an alpha receptor system.

Stimulants of the sympathetic nervous system (sympathomimetic drugs)

The action of the sympathetic nervous system can be enhanced at the nerve terminal, where norepinephrine is released, and at the alpha or beta adrenergic receptor sites on the effector cell (Fig. 18-1).

Alpha adrenergic stimulants

The alpha adrenergic stimulants are drugs that cause vasoconstriction and reflex vagal bradycardia. They are epinephrine (Adrenalin), norepinephrine (Levophed), methoxamine (Vasoxyl), and phenylephrine (Neo-Synephrine).

Beta adrenergic stimulants

The beta adrenergic stimulants are drugs that cause vasodilatation primarily in skeletal muscle. In the heart they cause accelerated conductivity, positive chronotropic and inotropic effects, increased cardiac output, and decreased end-systolic size. They are isoproterenol (Isuprel), epinephrine, norepinephrine, and isoxsuprine (Vasodilan).

Isoproterenol is a pure beta adrenergic stimulant. It is used in heart block because it stimulates the beta receptors in the ventricular conductive system. It is also a very potent positive inotropic agent.

Nerve terminal stimulants

The nerve terminal stimulants are drugs that cause norepinephrine to be released from the nerve ending, and consequently they have both alpha and beta effects. Examples are tyramine and ephedrine.

Antagonists of the sympathetic nervous system (sympatholytic drugs)

The action of the sympathetic nervous system can be blocked at three places (Fig. 18-1):

1 The adrenergic receptor (alpha or beta), where norepinephrine is received
2 The nerve terminal, where norepinephrine is released
3 The ganglion

Alpha adrenergic blocking agents

Alpha adrenergic blocking agents cause vascular dilatation, thus inducing a reduction in peripheral resistance and venous return as well as eliciting compensatory tachycardia. They are phenoxybenzamine (Dibenzyline), phentolamine (Regitine), ergot alkaloids (Hydergine), azapetine (Ilidar), chlorpromazine (Thorazine), and steroids in pharmacological doses.

Beta adrenergic blocking agents

Beta adrenergic blocking agents, because of their action on the beta receptor mechanism of the heart, have a marked negative inotropic effect. They are dichlorisoproterenol (DCI), pronethalol (Nethalide, Alderlin), propranolol (Inderal), and practolol.

Nerve terminal blocking agents

Nerve terminal blocking agents interfere with sympathetic nervous system activity by decreasing the available norepinephrine and therefore inhibiting both alpha and beta responses. This is accomplished by the following:

1 Preventing the release of norepinephrine (bretylium tosylate)
2 Inhibiting the synthesis of norepinephrine (methyltyrosine)
3 Depleting the nerve ending of norepinephrine (reserpine and guanethedine)

Ganglionic blocking agents

Both the sympathetic and parasympathetic systems are affected by these drugs since both systems have ganglia. They cause orthostatic hypotension, reduced venous return, and reduced peripheral resistance.

PARASYMPATHETIC NERVOUS SYSTEM

The parasympathetic nerve is composed of a preganglionic fiber, where acetylcholine is released; a cholinergic receptor, where acetylcholine is re-

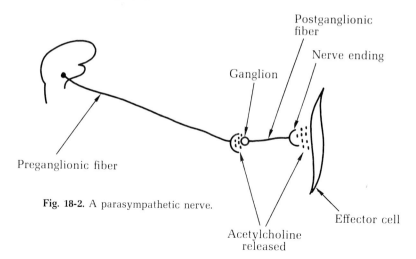

Fig. 18-2. A parasympathetic nerve.

ceived; a postganglionic fiber, where acetylcholine is again released; and cholinergic receptors located on the effector cell (end organ) (Fig. 18-2).

Parasympathetic function compared to sympathetic function

The vagus nerve supplies the parasympathetic innervation to the heart, mainly the atria. Thus these nerves (vagi) control the supraventricular functions of heart rate and A-V conduction.

Conversely, the ventricles are rich in sympathetic nerve innervation and poor in vagus innervation. Thus it is that the sympathetic nerves control ventricular function via the beta receptors. Therefore drugs blocking or stimulating the vagus nerve exert their effect almost entirely on the sinus and A-V nodes, enhancing or blocking rate and conduction. For example, atropine blocks the effects of the vagus nerve and has little effect on ventricular function.

By the same token, drugs blocking or stimulating the sympathetic nervous system affect the ventricles. For example, propranolol, a beta adrenergic blocking agent, markedly affects ventricular contractility and has only a moderate effect on the sinus or A-V nodes.

Terminology

acetylcholine Mediator of the parasympathetic nerve.

parasympathomimetic drugs (mimetic = mimic) Mimic the effects of stimuli to the parasympathetic nervous system.

cholinergic Refers to the receptors for acetylcholine or the parasympathomimetic drugs; these receptors are located in the ganglion and in the effector cell.

parasympatholytic drugs (Gr. lytikos = dissolving) Block or dissolve the effects of the parasympathetic nervous system.

cholinesterase An enzyme in the cholinergic receptors that is responsible for the breakdown or inactivation of acetylcholine.

cholinesterase inhibitors Enhance the effects of the parasympathetic nervous system by slowing the inactivation of acetylcholine, thus allowing the characteristic actions of the parasympathetic nervous system to proceed in an intensified manner; physostigmine (or eserine), neostigmine (Prostigmine), and edrophonium chloride (Tensilon) are examples.

Acetylcholine

As mediator of the parasympathetic nerve, acetylcholine has a negative chronotropic effect, decreasing the rate of the sinus node. It causes vasodilatation, which in turn elicits a reflex increase of sympathetic activity. There is therefore an increase in the heart rate and cardiac output as a compensatory activity.

Cholinergic blocking drugs

Cholinergic blocking drugs act by blocking the action of acetylcholine at the effector cell.

Atropine is this type of drug and causes an increase in heart rate and A-V conduction. The site of the action of atropine is directly on the effector cells and not on the nerve endings (Fig. 18-2). There it blocks the action of acetylcholine but not its liberation, thus reversing all of the effects of parasympathetic nervous stimulation. The heart rate is stimulated due to blockage of vagal effects on the sinus node.

ANTIARRHYTHMIC DRUGS
Digitalis

Digitalis has many modes of action. Its influence on the myocardium is complex and is affected by the autonomic nervous system.

Effects on the myocardium

Digitalis causes the atrial and ventricular tissues to become more excitable. Automaticity is enhanced, and conduction is slowed.

Effects on the action potential

At this point the reader is asked to review the discussion of the normal action potential in Chapter 2.

Digitalis causes the resting membrane potential to be reduced from -90 mv. to approximately -80 mv. The threshold at which excitation would take place is lowered, and the excitability of the heart is thus increased.

With the reduction in the resting membrane potential, there is also a reduction in the action potential (Fig. 18-3). The velocity of conduction is dependent upon these two values. Conduction is therefore slowed.

Phase 4 has a steeper slope, thus increasing automaticity (latent pacemaker activity is enhanced).

The positive inotropic effect of digitalis is due to the drug's ability to block the ATPase-supported sodium and potassium pumps. Potassium there-

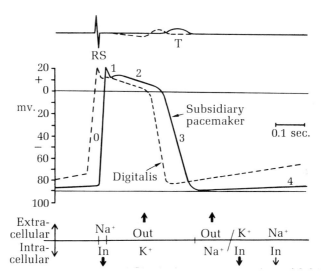

Fig. 18-3. Diagrammatic representation of the effect of digitalis on the action potential and the ECG (broken line). Bottom panel shows the transmembrane cation movement. (From Mason, D., Zelis, R., Lee, G., James, H., Spann, J., and Amsterdam, E.: Am. J. Cardiol. **27:**546, 1971.)

fore leaves the cell, and sodium enters, along with calcium. Thus calcium is directly provided during the contractile process, causing a stronger contraction.

The toxic effects of digitalis are due to an extension of the same phenomena, that is, to the increased automaticity of pacemaker tissues that occurs because of inhibition of the membrane pumps. The most common toxic effects are ectopics of the Purkinje system and A-V heart block. Bigeminy and multifocal ectopic beats are most often seen. Digitalis toxicity is enhanced by the presence of hypercalcemia.

Effects on the ECG

All of the ECG changes are directly related to the changes in the action potential (Fig. 18-3). The primary changes are a sagging of the S-T segment, so that it has a scooped appearance, and a shortening of the Q-T interval.

Quinidine

Quinidine is generally regarded as a myocardial depressant.

Effects on the myocardium

1 Pacemakers are depressed.
2 Automaticity is decreased.
3 Conduction velocity in the atria and ventricles is slowed.
4 Conduction velocity in the A-V junction is increased indirectly through the vagolytic action of quinidine.

Effects on the action potential

1 Quinidine decreases the slope of diastolic depolarization (phase 4) and thus decreases automaticity. Probably the most important therapeutic property of quinidine is that of abolishing ectopic impulse formation.
2 In higher doses, quinidine decreases the rate of rise of phase 0 and prolongs the action potential, thus slowing conduction, which is dependent upon the rate of rise of the action potential and its amplitude.
3 Phase 3 of the action potential is prolonged; thus the repolarization time is lengthened.

Effects on the ECG

1 QRS duration is prolonged.
2 Q-T interval is prolonged.
3 S-T deviation is induced.
4 There are T wave changes (increased duration, inversion, and notching) that are related to the action potential.
5 P wave duration is increased because of the prolonged atrial conduction time.

Toxicity

The most commonly cited toxic manifestation is diarrhea. Nausea and vomiting occur less frequently.

Quinidine syncope due to repetitive ventricular fibrillation has been estimated to occur in 3% to 4% of patients receiving high-dosage quinidine therapy.

The most serious toxic reaction is a decreasing rate of conduction through the myocardium, resulting finally in intraventricular block. This toxic effect is indicated by a broadening of the QRS complex.

Procainamide hydrochloride (Pronestyl)

Procainamide hydrochloride is a derivative of procaine. It has a quinidine-like action in that it depresses the myocardium by decreasing the slope of diastolic depolarization (phase 4) and lengthening repolarization (the terminal portion of phase 3). Thus it makes the heart less able to respond to ectopic stimuli. Procainamide hydrochloride sometimes slows A-V conduction and prolongs intraventricular conduction time.

Lidocaine hydrochloride (Xylocaine)

In contrast to procainamide hydrochloride and quinidine, lidocaine hydrochloride has no significant effects on A-V conduction or intraventricular conduction and has a less depressant effect on myocardial contraction since it does not affect phase 0 or membrane responsiveness. It acts mainly by suppressing phase 4. It also shortens the action potential and effective refractory period.

Diphenylhydantoin (Dilantin)

Diphenylhydantoin increases the rate of rise of the action potential, thus improving conduction in those fibers via a slow rate of rise in phase 0. Diphenylhydantoin also decreases the slope of diastolic depolarization (phase 4), thus depressing ventricular automaticity. It also shortens repolarization time (phase 3).

If these effects are compared to the effect of digitalis on the action potential, it becomes apparent that diphenyldantoin is a valuable drug in the treatment of digitalis toxicity.

ELECTROLYTES

With an understanding of the processes involved in maintaining the resting membrane potential in the single cell, we reach some appreciation of the importance of electrolyte balance in the body. It is through the action of ions on the cell membrane that the depolarization process takes place and electrochemical currents are transmitted within the muscle fibers.

Potassium

Potassium (K^+) is found in abundance in the body. Because of this, and because of the ease with which this ion diffuses across the cell membrane, it plays a major role in maintaining the integrity of the cell.

It is excreted by the body in the urine, feces, and perspiration. Therefore diuretics as well as vomiting, diaphoresis, and diarrhea can rapidly deplete the body of this vital ion. An abnormally low potassium content of the blood is called hypokalemia.

Conversely, anuria can cause a potassium buildup, creating an abnormally high potassium concentration (hyperkalemia). Both hyperkalemia and hypokalemia may produce serious arrhythmias and death.

Hyperkalemia

The resting membrane potential is dependent for its strength on the size of the potassium gradient across the membrane. In its resting state there is approximately thirty times as much K^+ within the cell as there is in the extracellular fluid. The action potential is dependent on the strength of the resting membrane potential for its amplitude, or the amount of positive overshoot, and for the rate of rise of this amplitude. Conduction velocity is in turn dependent upon rapid depolarization. Neighboring fibers are stimulated faster by a strong action potential with a steep rise (phase 0).

In summary, the resting membrane potential, the action potential, and conduction velocity are all dependent for their strength and speed on the potassium gradient.

Hyperkalemia (elevated levels of extracellular K^+) causes the gradient of that ion across the cell membrane to be lessened. This causes the resting

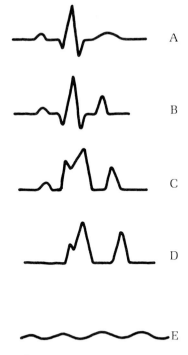

Fig. 18-4. ECG changes in hyperkalemia. See text for explanation.

membrane potential to be lowered, and this in turn reduces the action potential and slows conduction. The characteristic effect of hyperkalemia is therefore slow conduction (intra-atrial, atrioventricular, and/or intraventricular heart block).

ECG CHANGES

1 The normal serum K^+ is 4 to 5.5 mEq. per liter (Fig. 18-4, *A*).
2 Changes start early (K^+ 6 mEq. per liter), with a peaked T wave and a normal QRS complex and P-R interval (Fig. 18-4, *B*).
3 The QRS widens and is slurred (K^+ 7 to 7.5 mEq. per liter) (Fig. 18-4, *C*).
4 Atrial conduction ceases and the P wave is not seen. The broad QRS persists (K^+ 8 mEq. per liter) (Fig. 18-4, *D*).
5 The sine (curved) wave is seen as a terminal event (Fig. 18-4, *E*).

Hypokalemia

The effects of hypokalemia are mainly the result of loss of the potassium gradient across the cell membrane and the effect of this loss on the action potential. Automaticity is increased, and there is an interference with the normal repolarization process, causing ectopic beats and changes in the S-T segment and T wave.

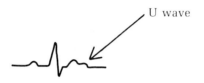

Fig. 18-5. U wave seen in hypokalemia.

There is a prominent U wave (a positive deflection immediately following or at the end of the T wave). The Q-T interval often appears prolonged due to the superimposition of the U wave on the T. The true Q-T interval is of normal duration in hypokalemia (Fig. 18-5). ·

Calcium

The level of myocardial contractility is thought to be determined by the number of calcium ions available. There are four proteins involved in the process of myocardial contraction: myosin, actin, tropomyosin, and troponin. Contraction is inhibited by the combination of troponin-tropomyosin. The contractile process is initiated when calcium, released by excitation of the cell membrane, becomes bound to troponin. Therefore calcium has a direct effect on myocardial contractility. Increased extracellular calcium improves cardiac contractility. In levels exceeding the body's tolerance it would produce rigor of the myocardium.

ECG changes due to hypercalcemia are so slight as to be of no diagnostic value. In hypocalcemia, repolarization is prolonged, causing a duration of the Q-T interval that is beyond normal limits.

TEST TRACINGS

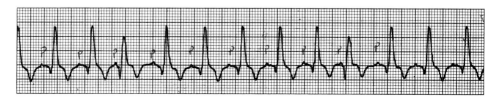

Fig. 18-6

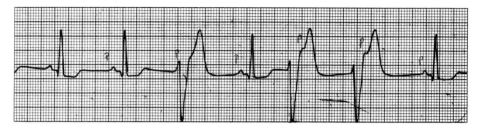

Fig. 18-7

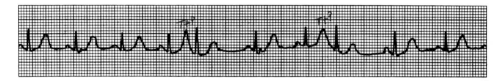

Fig. 18-8

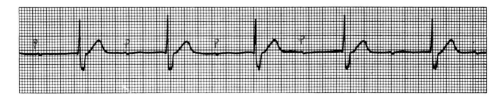

Fig. 18-9

ANSWERS

18-6 *Sinus tachycardia with PACs.* The two PACs in this tracing are only very slightly premature (0.02 second). They are slightly narrower and more peaked than the sinus P waves and are followed by aberrant ventricular conduction (a deeper S and shorter R). The sinus rate is 106.

18-7 *Frequent, unifocal PVCs.* The identical contour of these PVCs make it evident that they are generated by the same ectopic focus.

18-8 *PACs.* The P' waves distort the preceding T wave and are both followed by normal ventricular conduction.

18-9 *First-degree heart block.* The P-R interval is a full second. The P wave is a small biphasic deflection. Since the QRS interval is also prolonged, the conduction defect involves the bundle branches.

19 Electrical hazards of ECG monitoring

The explosive growth in the use of electronic medical diagnostic instrumentation has unfortunately not been accompanied by a similar growth in awareness of the electrical shock hazards that may be present. Current trends indicate that more rather than less instrumentation will be used in the future, for these instruments provide the physician with powerful analytical tools to help determine the course of treatment. In this context it is imperative that a greater effort be made to minimize the possibility of electrical shock to the patient. There are four main areas that affect patient safety:

1 Equipment design
2 Unit power installation
3 Nursing technique
4 Periodic inspection and maintenance

Coordinated efforts in all of these areas will result in a high level of patient safety.

The primary reason for the increased shock hazard is the use of catheters that provide a direct electrical connection to the myocardium. This creates what we will refer to as the "electrically sensitive patient." Because the cardiac tissue is directly exposed, the patient is susceptible to a level of electrical shock that an uncatheterized person cannot perceive. In order to fully appreciate the susceptibility of the electrically sensitive patient, an understanding of the nature of electrical current flow and its relationship to applied voltage and path resistance is necessary.

ALTERNATING CURRENT (AC) FLOW

The power used for operating electrical equipment within the hospital is 120 volt, 60 Hertz AC. This power is available at the standard three-pin wall receptacle and is connected to the equipment in use by means of the usual three-pronged plug and line cord (Fig. 19-1).

The longer round pin is the grounding or ground pin and plays an important part in patient safety. One of the flat blades is the "hot" connecting pin and the other is the "neutral" connecting pin. This terminology is different from that used for the depolarizing current that occurs within the heart in that the positive (+) and negative (−) symbols are not used. This is because the "hot" is constantly changing from positive to negative and back again, while the "neutral" is changing from negative to positive and back. The two are always out of step (one is positive while the other is negative), so that the resultant current flow is constantly changing or *alternating* in direction, hence the term "alternating current." These alternations take place sixty times a second. However, in the discussion of patient safety this instantaneous

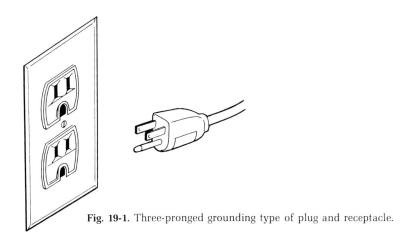

Fig. 19-1. Three-pronged grounding type of plug and receptacle.

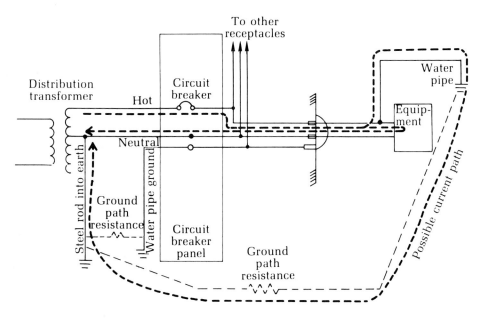

Fig. 19-2. Normal and ground current paths.

current flow is of little concern, and the current flow will be considered to be the usual AC concept in which current flows from the "hot" to the "neutral."

In the normal system of power distribution the neutral is connected to ground. This creates another path for current flow, that of hot to ground (Fig. 19-2).

Ground

The earth itself is a conductor of electricity, albeit a poor one. Its conductivity is due to the moisture and resultant ions in the soil and an extensive network of conductive metal water pipes, gas pipes, conduits, and so on. While it is true that a relatively high resistance exists between a water pipe and a short rod driven into the earth, it is also true that a low resistance exists between points served by the same water main, even though they are in different buildings. A conductive rod that is driven into the ground so that it contacts the moist soil that lies under the surface will also exhibit a relatively low resistance to a water pipe. The result is a conductive network of pipes, ground water, and conduits that connects users of electricity. It is this network that is referred to as ground.

It is obvious that, if only for safety reasons, the power distribution system must take this ground network into account. The method used is one in which the distribution transformer develops 240 volts alternating current (vac). A center tap on the transformer allows half of the voltage (120 vac) to be made available. Although 120 vac is supplied for most equipment, 240 vac is supplied for heavier equipment such as pumps, compressors, and air conditioners. The transformer center tap is connected to ground, thereby establishing the hot side of the line at 120 vac above ground. This grounding prevents the hot side of the line from exceeding 120 vac, thus providing the maximum practical safety for the voltage involved. Still, dangerous currents can flow from the hot side of the line to any ground. It is this additional path that is responsible for a preponderance of electrical shock hazard.

Ohm's law

The relationship between the applied voltage, path resistance, and resultant current flow is known as Ohm's law. Mathematically the relationship is represented by the following equation:

$$\text{Current (I)} = \frac{\text{Voltage (V)}}{\text{Resistance (R)}}$$

Briefly, this expression states that the current flow increases as the applied voltage is increased and decreases as the circuit path resistance is increased. The units of measurement involved are volts, the unit of voltage; ohms, the unit of resistance; and amperes (amp.), the unit of current. The usual scaling prefixes such as milli- (1/1000), micro- (1/1,000,000), kilo- (1000), and mega- (1,000,000) are used with these units. Just as a milligram is one-thousandth

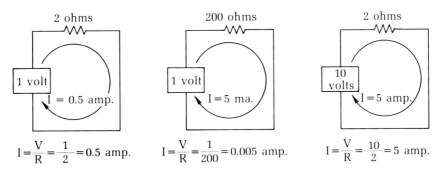

Fig. 19-3. Effect of changing resistance and voltage on current flow.

of a gram, a milliampere (ma.) is one-thousandth of an ampere. The prefixes kilo- and mega-, for the purposes of this discussion, apply only to resistance. The examples in Fig. 19-3 illustrate the effect of changing resistance and voltage on current flow.

ELECTRICAL SHOCK

As discussed in previous chapters, the operation of the heart is dependent upon precisely timed, internally generated electrical pulses. The effect of electrical shock is to disrupt the coordinated contraction and relaxation of the cardiac muscle and cause ventricular fibrillation. In cases of very severe shock the heart is completely stopped by sustained contraction. The severity of an electrical shock is related to the current flow through the tissue involved. The shock can vary from an intensity that is almost imperceptible to one that is fatal. Various studies have been made on the effect of electrical shock on both humans and dogs, and the results of some of these studies are summarized in Table 1.

Macroshock

Gross electrical shock is the type in which the current passes through the trunk, and contact to the source is made through intact skin. In this situation the current spreads throughout all of the tissue in its path, and the amount of current that flows through cardiac tissue is a very small fraction of the total. The intact skin exhibits a resistance to the current that ranges from 1000 ohms (for conditions of good contact and moist skin) to more than 1,000,000 ohms (1 megohm) (for dry skin and low relative humidity).

The body has two defenses against electrical shock. First, the high resistance of the skin reduces the amount of current that can flow due to a given impressed voltage (Ohm's law). Therefore contact with even full 110-volt line voltage generally results in a painful but nonfatal shock. Second, as we have pointed out, there is a spreading effect whereby the current is dis-

Table 1. Effect of shock current on the heart

Current	Through intact skin	Direct contact to myocardium
10 amp.	Sustained myocardial contraction	
5 amp.		
2 amp.		
1 amp.		
500 ma.	Ventricular fibrillation	
200 ma.	(respiration continues)	
100 ma.		
50 ma.	Pain, fainting, exhaustion	
20 ma.		
10 ma.	"Let go" current	
5 ma.	Maximum harmless current	Ventricular fibrillation (humans)
2 ma.		(2.5 cm. diam. plate electrode)
1 ma.	Threshold of perception	
500 μa.		Ventricular fibrillation (humans)
200 μa.		(0.25 cm. diam. plate electrode)
100 μa.		
50 μa.		Ventricular fibrillation in dogs
20 μa.		(catheter)
10 μa.		Maximum current recommended for
5 μa.		electrically safe areas

tributed throughout the tissue in its path. Because of this spreading, the cardiac tissue is exposed to only a small fraction of the current passing through the body.

Taking these protective mechanisms into account, electrical safety standards have been established and implemented. Of these many standards, that pertaining to leakage currents is of particular relevance to this discussion and is identified in Table 1. The success of these standards is demonstrated by the fact that despite the extensive use of electrical equipment, serious shock due to normal use of modern equipment in good repair is very rare. However effective these standards have been for the protection of the uncatheterized person, they are not adequate to ensure the safety of the electrically sensitive patient. To protect these patients, more stringent standards must be met.

Microshock

The electrically sensitive patient is susceptible to current levels that are imperceptible to the normal person. Studies have shown that ventricular fibrillation can be induced in a catheterized patient with current levels below 1 ma. (Table 1). This greatly increased vulnerability of the electrically sensitive patient to electrical shock is due to the broaching of the body's two defenses. First, the use of a catheter can reduce the path resistance from the normal 1-megohm to 1000-ohm range to a range of from 500 to 1000 ohms.

Second, and more critical, is the ineffectiveness of the current-spreading effect that, in the case of a shock across the trunk, diminishes the amount of current flowing through the cardiac tissue. While it is still true that the current is distributed through the tissue in its path, the catheter makes a direct connection with the myocardium, so that all of the tissue in the current path is cardiac tissue.

Due to the extremely small currents involved in the microshock environment, a potentially lethal condition can exist and not be perceived by uncatheterized persons coming into contact with the current source. As can be seen in Table 1, the imperceptible current of 1 ma. can cause fibrillation. It is this inability of operating personnel to determine when a dangerous condition exists that makes a periodic inspection program necessary to ensure patient safety.

SOURCES OF CURRENTS

After discussing the nature of AC microcurrent flow and its effect on the electrically sensitive patient, a question arises as to the origin of these currents. Once the sources of these dangerous currents are known, steps may be taken to locate and eliminate them.

Leakage currents

The most probable source of currents dangerous to the electrically sensitive patient is what are generally referred to as leakage currents. While the term suggests that some sort of malfunction must exist in a piece of electrical equipment in order for it to "leak" current, the leakage is in fact due to a normal electrical characteristic known as capacitive coupling. Whenever an AC voltage is impressed between two electrical conductors that are in close proximity, a current will flow through the conductors, even though they are perfectly insulated from each other. This characteristic of coupling AC current through an insulator is what is known as capacitive coupling. The amount of current flow depends on several parameters. Among these are the amount of separation between the conductors (the less the separation, the greater the current flow), the effective area of the conductors (the greater the common area, the greater the current flow), and impressed voltage (the greater the impressed voltage, the greater the current flow).

A moment's reflection on capacitive coupling will show that an entire spectrum of potential current paths has been opened. For the types and sizes of equipment in use in the unit, these capacitive leakage currents are small and harmless to operating personnel and patients who are not electrically sensitive. However, the electrically sensitive patient is susceptible to these current levels.

The amount of leakage current can and does increase when the equipment is subjected to a humid environment, moisture, spillage, dust, or a corrosive atmosphere. These cause the deterioration of insulation used in the equipment and consequently lower the insulation resistance. This type of leakage is known as resistance leakage. It is different from but can occur in addition to the capacitive leakage discussed earlier. The result is that the two leakages add and increase the shock hazard, at times to the point at which the equipment is hazardous even to the nonelectrically sensitive person. Equipment such as vacuum cleaners, floor waxers, and pumps that is subject to adverse environmental conditions can develop high-leakage currents.

The usual method of protecting the user from leakage currents is to ground, by means of the grounding pin on the plug, the case or housing of the equipment.

Equipment faults

Faults (shorts) are actual malfunctions of the equipment whereby a wire comes in contact with another wire or with the case. The situation that causes a shock hazard is a fault to the case or housing. Depending upon the point in the circuit at which the fault occurs, the voltage on the case can range from 120 volts to a few millivolts.

The method of protection here is the same as for leakage currents, that is, grounding the case by means of a three-pin power plug. The fault current is then conducted harmlessly to ground. It is obvious that if the fault current were large the circuit breaker or fuse supplying the current would open, interrupting the current and publicizing the malfunction. What is not obvious is that substantial current can flow without opening the circuit breaker or fuse, because circuit breakers or fuses are designed to carry 15 to 20 amp. without opening. If the total of normal current and fault current does not exceed this rating, no opening will occur. In many instances the faulty equipment will continue to operate normally or give a slightly degraded performance. However, if the grounding circuit should ever be broken, a hazard is present for the electrically sensitive patient that could also affect the operating personnel.

This ground connection is the mainstay of patient safety. However, it is effective only to the extent that it provides an extremely low resistance path to a true ground. Hence it is necessary that a well-designed grounding system be used and maintained in the areas where patients are susceptible to microshock.

TYPICAL HAZARDOUS SITUATIONS

After investigating the sources of potentially dangerous currents and determining the levels of current that can be a threat to the electrically sensitive patient, it is helpful to explore potentially dangerous situations that may arise in the cardiac care unit.

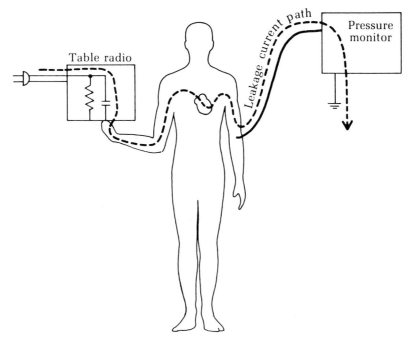

Fig. 19-4. Leakage current path for ungrounded equipment.

Ungrounded equipment

Ungrounded equipment can be readily identified by its use of a two-pronged rather than a three-pronged plug. The two-pronged plug has no provision for routing any leakage or fault current safely to the power grounding system. If a piece of ungrounded equipment is defective, it can pose a hazard to the nonelectrically sensitive patient and operating personnel as well as to the electrically sensitive patient. When operating normally and in good repair, ungrounded equipment is still a hazard to the electrically sensitive patient. Take, for example, the patient who has a pacemaker or an indwelling catheter for cardiac pressure monitoring. The catheter, through its associated monitor, provides a resistance to ground that is sufficiently low to allow the leakage current of an ungrounded table radio to pass through the heart if contact is made with the conductive case of the radio (Fig. 19-4).

Equipment with a defective ground

The hazards posed by equipment with open or defective grounding systems are similar to those posed by ungrounded equipment. Although ungrounded equipment can be readily identified and removed, the identification of equipment with an open ground is not as easy. A visual inspection of power cords is helpful, but to ensure patient safety, a resistance measurement must be made of all grounds.

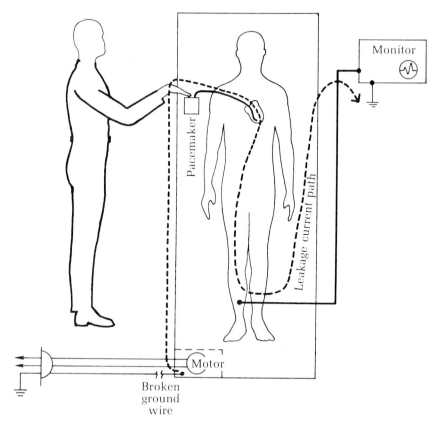

Fig. 19-5. Attendant as part of leakage current path.

As in the previous case of a grounded pressure catheter, a defective ground on an electric bed would allow a dangerous current to flow through the patient's heart if an attendant were to touch the bare pacemaker terminal while holding the bed rail (Fig. 19-5).

Unequal ground potentials

Throughout most of the previous discussion one ground was considered to be the same as any other, at least within the cardiac care unit. To ensure patient safety, it is necessary that the various grounds associated with a given patient be at, or at least very close to, the same electrical potential. Failure to meet this requirement will allow a current to pass through the patient if he is connected to two pieces of equipment that are connected to two different grounds. For example, if a patient were connected to a pressure monitor transducer that is normally grounded and to an electrocardiograph machine that has the usual right-leg ground, a current due to the difference in ground potentials could flow through his heart (Fig. 19-6).

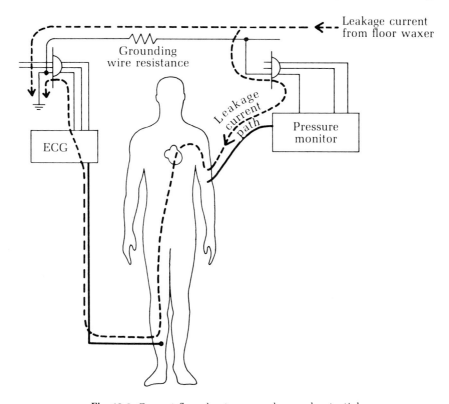

Fig. 19-6. Current flow due to unequal ground potentials.

The detection of potential differences between receptacle grounds is made more difficult because the potential is usually due to a high-leakage current flowing through the ground system. This leakage current may come from equipment that is not in the unit. In addition, the equipment causing the leakage current may not be in continuous operation, with the result that the difference in ground potentials varies.

WHAT CAN BE DONE

Paramount to achieving a safe environment for the electrically sensitive patient is the establishment of an electrically safe area. Within this area, special precautions should be enforced with regard to plant wiring, equipment that is allowed, inspection and maintenance procedures, and training of personnel.

Plant wiring

In the electrically safe area all receptacles must be of the three-pin grounding type. The technique of using the wiring conduit or a small-gauge wire for grounding purposes is inadequate for this area. A separate twelve-

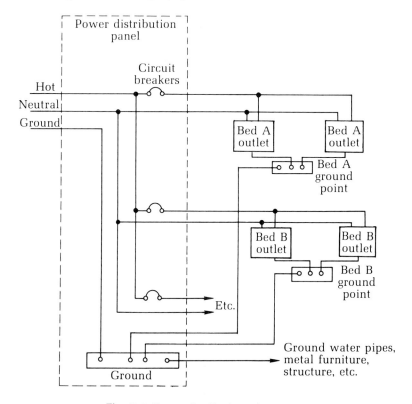

Fig. 19-7. Power distribution scheme.

gauge wire should be used for ground. To equalize the grounds at a given bed at the same potential, all the ground wires from outlets serving that bed should be grounded at a single point, and that ground should not connect to outlets other than those serving that bed. All exposed metal items such as water pipes, building structure, and metal furniture must be connected to a room ground (Fig. 19-7).

If equipment that grounds or is likely to ground indwelling electrodes is used, it is advisable to investigate the use of isolation transformers for the area. Isolation transformers provide an additional margin of safety for patients in the case of grounding failures.

Equipment selection

Equipment used for ECG monitoring has continually improved with respect to features that enhance both diagnostic usefulness and patient safety. Early ECG monitors that used a grounded input posed a hazard if the potential between the electrically sensitive patient and the monitor exceeded 10 mv. The later development of the driven right-leg circuits provided patient protection for voltages up to 500 mv. Since typical voltages that result in differences in ground potentials seldom exceed 1 volt, a measure of protection from this hazard is afforded the patient.

The ECG monitor with isolated input circuitry has input amplifiers that are greatly isolated from the rest of the monitor. This is accomplished by means of special circuitry that supplies operating power to the input amplifier and couples the signal to the display on the scope. As a result, the patient is protected against hazardous currents even though the potential between the patient and monitor is full-line voltage (120 volts). The patient would thus be protected in the case of a broken grounding wire.

Telemetry techniques are used in some ECG monitors. In this type of equipment the input amplifier and a telemetry transmitter are combined in a small unit that is worn by the patient. The entire patient unit is powered by a battery, so that complete isolation from the power lines and their attendant hazards is provided. The patient unit sends out a radio signal that is received by the monitor and displayed. Such a system allows the patient to be ambulatory.

The responsibility for a final decision as to the selection of new equipment and other capital improvements usually rests with hospital administrators whose primary field of expertise is, in a broad sense, business management. In order to make rational decisions regarding equipment, administrators must either gain expertise in this technical field or seek outside counsel. The latter course is usually the most efficient. Needless to say, the consultant should be both technically competent and unbiased. He should be made aware of the hospital's insistence on a safe environment for the electrically sensitive patient.

Personnel training

While it is certainly true that proper wiring and equipment play an important part in determining patient safety in the electrically safe area, all personnel working within this area must be made aware of the acute vulnerability of the electrically sensitive patient.

With regard to patient safety, the first task of personnel working within the cardiac care unit or other electrically safe areas is to avoid becoming part of a circuit that could allow current to flow through them and then through the patient. Pressure catheters, intracardiac electrodes, and pacing catheters provide direct electrical connections to the patient's heart. It is important that all metal terminals, guide wires, and uninsulated electrode wires be insulated to prevent contact with either personnel or ground. This insulation can be provided by placing plastic or rubber sleeving over exposed terminals, wearing surgical gloves whenever it is necessary to handle bare electrode wires or terminals, and placing external battery-powered pacemakers in a surgical glove or plastic sheet to insulate their terminals. When taking an intracardiac ECG, it is imperative that the intracardiac electrode be connected to lead V and not to the indifferent (right-leg) electrode.

The second task is that of maintaining a continuing survey of the condition of equipment within the unit. If a tingling sensation (mild electrical shock) is felt when a piece of equipment is touched, it is an indication that the equipment is defective and poses a definite shock hazard to the patient. If not required for life support of the patient, the equipment should be removed from the area and tagged to alert others to the danger. When it is required for life support, the equipment should be repaired as soon as possible or replaced with a similar item.

The condition of all power cords and plugs should be noted. The hospital electrician should repair or replace all frayed or damaged cords. Any equipment using two-pronged plugs should be removed from the unit until they can be replaced with the three-pronged grounding type. Care should be taken to avoid damaging power cords by running heavy wheeled equipment over them or storing them in a manner that exposes them to kinking or extremes of temperature.

Appearance of AC interference on the ECG tracing can be due to several causes. Some of these pose a hazard to the patient; others do not. In either event the interference makes the tracing difficult to interpret, and the situation should be corrected at once. Check the patient cables and ensure that the electrodes have not dried out. If this does not correct the problem, it is possible that AC currents are flowing through the patient cable. The source of the interference should be found and corrected as soon as possible.

Inspection

To maintain a continuing high level of patient safety, it is necessary to initiate a system of periodic inspections. These inspections must cover both the electrically safe area and any equipment that may be brought into it. The main object of the inspection is to ensure that none of the equipment can subject the patient to a current of greater than 10 microamperes (μa.). As shown in Table 1, the accepted maximum safe current level for an electrically sensitive patient has been established at 10 μa.

The amount of current a patient could receive can be determined by measuring the voltage across a 500-ohm resistor (that simulates the resistance of the patient) connected between the case of an instrument and true ground. This measurement is repeated for all metal surfaces and terminals in the electrically safe area. Ohm's law is used to determine the maximum allowable voltage corresponding to a current of 10 μa. and a resistance of 500 ohms. When these parameters are substituted in the equation $V = I \times R$, a value of 5 mv. is obtained. Additional measurements should be made to ensure that all receptacle grounds are within 5 mv. of each other. Although the measurements described are relatively straightforward, special equipment, fixtures, and techniques are required. Unless the hospital is large enough to maintain this equipment and expertise, outside professional assistance should be engaged.

REFERENCES

BOOKS

Beckwith, J.: Grant's clinical electrocardiography, the spatial vector approach, New York, 1970, McGraw-Hill Book Co., Inc.

Berne, R. M., and Levy, M. N.: Cardiovascular physiology, St. Louis, 1967, The C. V. Mosby Co.

Friedberg, C. K.: Diseases of the heart, ed. 3, Philadelphia, 1966, W. B. Saunders Co.

Moran, N.: Beta adrenergic blockage, an historical review and evaluation. In Kattus, A. A., Ross, G., and Hall, V. E., editors: Cardiovascular beta adrenergic responses, Berkeley, 1970, University of California Press.

Sano, T., Mizuhira, V., and Matsuda, K.: Electrophysiology and ultrastructure of the heart, New York, 1967, Grune & Stratton, Inc.

Stock, J. P.: Diagnosis and treatment of cardiac arrhythmias, London, 1969, Butterworth & Co.

JOURNAL ARTICLES

AAMI outlines steps to help protect patients from electrical hazards, Hosp. Top. **49:**84, 1971.

Abildskov, J., Millar, K., and Burgess, M.: Atrial fibrillation, Am. J. Cardiol. **28:**263, 1971.

Attwood, P.: Follow these four steps to electrical safety, Mod. Hosp. **116:**64, 1971.

Barold, S., and Linhart, J.: Recent advances in the treatment of ectopic tachycardia by electrical pacing, Am. J. Cardiol. **25:**698, 1970.

Boinear, J., and Moore, N.: Evidence for propagation of activation across an accessory atrio-ventricular connection in type A and B pre-excitation, Circulation **41:**375, 1970.

Breller, B., Kotler, M., and Collens, R.: The use of ventricular pacing for suppression of ectopic ventricular activity, Am. J. Cardiol. **25:**467, 1970.

Bruner, J.: Hazards of electrical apparatus, Anesthesiology **28:**396, 1967.

Castellanos, A., Castillo, C., Agha, A., and Tressler, M.: His bundle electrograms in patients with short P-R intervals, narrow QRS complexes and paroxysmal tachycardia, Circulation **43:**667, 1971.

Castellanos, A., Maytin, O., Lemberg, L., and Castillo, C.: Unusual QRS complexes produced by pacemaker stimuli, Am. Heart J. **77:**732, 1969.

Castillo, C., and Castellanos, A.: His bundle recordings in patients with reciprocating tachycardias and Wolff-Parkinson-White syndrome, Circulation **42:**271, 1970.

Castillo, C., Maytin, O., and Castellanos, A.: His bundle recordings in atypical A-V nodal Wenckebach block during cardiac pacing, Am. J. Cardiol. **27:**570, 1971.

Castellanos, A., and Spence, M.: Pacemaker arrhythmias in context, Am. J. Cardiol. **25:**372, 1970.

Cole, J., Wills, R., Winterscheid, L., Reichenbach, D., and Blackmon, J.: The Wolff-Parkinson-White syndrome, problems in evaluation and surgical therapy, Circulation **42:**111, 1970.

Danzig, R., Alpern, H., and Swan, H.: The significance of atrial rate in patients with atrioventricular conduction abnormalities complicating acute myocardial infarction, Am. J. Cardiol. **24:**707, 1969.

Dreifus, L., Watanabe, Y., Haiat, R., and Kimbiris, D.: Atrioventricular block, Am. J. Cardiol. **28:**371, 1971.

181

Durrer, D., Schuilenburg, R., and Wellens, H.: Pre-excitation revisited, Am. J. Cardiol. **25**:690, 1970.

Dye, C.: Atrial tachycardia in Wolff-Parkinson-White syndrome, Am. J. Cardiol. **24**:265, 1969.

Fernandez, F., Scebat, L., and Lenegre, J.: Electrocardiographic study of left intraventricular hemiblock in man during selective coronary arteriography, Am. J. Cardiol. **26**:1, 1970.

Fisch, C., Greenspan, K., and Anderson, G.: Exit block, Am. J. Cardiol. **28**:402, 1971.

Gersony, W., and Ekery, D.: Concealed right bundle branch block in the presence of type B ventricular pre-excitation, Am. Heart J. **77**:668, 1969.

Goldreyer, B., and Damato, A.: Essential role of atrioventricular conduction delay in the initiation of paroxysmal supraventricular tachycardia, Circulation **43**:679, 1971.

Han, J.: Mechanisms of ventricular arrhythmias associated with myocardial infarction, Am. J. Cardiol **24**:800, 1961.

Han, J.: The concepts of reentrant activity responsible for ectopic rhythms, Am. J. Cardiol. **28**:253, 1971.

James, T.: Pathogenesis of arrhythmias in acute myocardial infarction, Am. J. Cardiol. **24**:791, 1969.

Kaplan, M., and Cohen, K.: Ventricular fibrillation in the Wolff-Parkinson-White syndrome, Am. J. Cardiol. **24**:259, 1969.

Kastor, J., Berkivite, B., and DeSanctis, R.: Variations in discharge rate of demand pacemakers not due to malfunction, Am. J. Cardiol. **25**:344, 1970.

Kelly, D.: Comparison of right atrial and right ventricular single and paired pacing in the canine heart, Am. Heart J. **77**:206, 1961.

Lasseter, K.: Treatment of arrhythmias: basic considerations, Med. Clin. North Am. **55**:435, 1971.

Lemberg, L., Castellanos, A., and Arcebal, A.: The vectorcardiogram in acute left anterior hemiblock, Am. J. Cardiol. **28**:483, 1971.

Marriott, H., and Hogan, P.: Hemiblock in acute myocardial infarction, Chest **58**:342, 1970.

Mason, D., Zelis, R., Lee, G., Hughes, J., Spann, J., and Amsterdam, E.: Current concepts and treatment of digitalis toxicity, Am. J. Cardiol. **27**:546, 1971.

Massumi, R., and Rice, J.: Incomplete bilateral bundle branch block, Am. J. Cardiol. **24**:890, 1969.

McNally, E., and Benchimol, A.: Medical and physiological considerations in the use of artificial cardiac pacing, Am. Heart J. **75**:380, 679, 1968.

Moore, W., Knoebel, S., and Spear, J.: Concealed conduction, Am. J. Cardiol. **28**:406, 1971.

Moran, N.: Adrenergic receptors, drugs and the cardiovascular system, Mod. Concepts Cardiovasc. Dis. **35**:93, 1966.

Moran, N.: The role of alpha and beta adrenergic receptors in the control of the circulation and in the actions of drugs on the cardiovascular system, Publication No. 942, Atlanta, 1971, Division of Basic Health Sciences, Emory University.

Narula, O., and Scherlag, B.: Analysis of the A-V conduction defect in complete heart block utilizing His bundle electrograms, Circulation **41**:437, 1970.

Narula, O., and Samet, P.: Wenckebach and Mobitz Type II A-V block due to block within the His bundle and bundle branches, Circulation **41**:947, 1970.

Narula, O., Cohen, L., Samet, P., Lister, J., Scherlag, B., and Hildner, F.: Localization of A-V conduction defects in man by recording of the His bundle electrogram, Am. J. Cardiol. **25**:228, 1970.

Okel, B.: The Wolff-Parkinson-White syndrome, Am. Heart J. **75**:673, 1968.

Parsonnet, V., Myers, G., Gilbert, L., and Zucker, R.: Prediction of impending pacemaker failure in a pacemaker clinic, Am. J. Cardiol. **25**:311, 1970.

Pruitt, R.: Ventricular pre-excitation (Wolff-Parkinson-White syndrome), Am. J. Cardiol. **25**:734, 1970.

Rosen, K., Rahimtoola, S., Chuquimia, R., Loeb, H., and Gunnar, R.: Electrophysiological significance of first degree atrioventricular block with intraventricular conduction disturbance, Circulation **43**:491, 1971.

Rosselot, E., Ahumada, J., Spoerer, A., and Sepulveda, G.: Trifascicular block treated by artificial pacing, Am. J. Cardiol. **26**:6, 1970.

Rosenbaum, M., Elizari, M., Lazzari, J., Nau, G., Levi, R., and Halpern, M.: Intraventricular trifascicular blocks. The syndrome of right bundle branch block with intermittent left anterior and posterior hemiblock, Am. Heart J. **78**:306, 1969.

Rosenbaum, M., Elizari, M., Lazzari, J., Nau, G., Levi, R., and Halpern, M.: Intraventricular trifascicular blocks. Review of the literature and classification, Am. Heart J. **78**:450, 1969.

Rosenbaum, M., Elizari, M., Levi, R., Nau, G., Pisani, N., Lazzari, J., and Halpern, M.: Five cases of intermittent left anterior hemiblock, Am. J. Cardiol. **24**:1, 1969.

Rothfeld, E., Zucker, I., Parsonnet, V., and Bernstein, A.: Paired pacing after coronary artery ligation, Am. J. Cardiol. **23**:224, 1969.

Sano, T., Suzuki, R., and Tsuchihashi, H.: Function of potential bypass tracts for atrioventricular conduction, Circulation **41**:413, 1970.

Scherf, D.: The mechanism of sinoatrial block, Am. J. Cardiol. **23**:769, 1969.

Scherlag, B., Lau, S., Helfant, R., Berkowitz, W., Stein, E., and Damato, A.: Catheter technique for recording His bundle activity in man, Circulation **39**:13, 1969.

Singer, D., and Fick, E. T.: Aberrancy: electrophysiologic aspects, Am. J. Cardiol. **28**:381, 1971.

Staewen, W., Lubin, D., Mower, M., and Tabatznik, B.: The significance of leakage currents in hospital electrical devices, Mt. Sinai J. Med. **15**:3, 1969.

Stanley, P.: Electrical shock hazards, Hospitals **45**:58, 73, 1971.

Starmer, C., Whalen, R., and McIntosh, H.: Hazards of electric shock in cardiology, Am. J. Cardiol. **14**:537, 1964.

Steiner, C., Sun, L., Stein, E., Wit, W., Weiss, M., Damato, A., Haft, J., Weinstock, M., and Prem, G.: Electrophysiologic documentation of trifascicular block as the common cause of complete heart block, Am. J. Cardiol. **28**:436, 1971.

Surawicz, B.: Ventricular fibrillation, Am. J. Cardiol. **28**:268, 1971.

Von Der Mosel, H.: Electrical safety and our hospitals, J. Assoc. Advance. Med. Instrument. **4**:2, 1970.

Vassalle, M.: Automaticity and automatic rhythms, Am. J. Cardiol. **28**:245, 1971.

Wellens, H., Shuilenberg, R., and Surrer, D.: Electrical stimulation of the heart in patients with Wolff-Parkinson-White syndrome, Type A, Circulation **43**:99, 1971.

INDEX*

A

Aberrant ventricular conduction; see Conduction, aberrant ventricular
AC; see Alternating current
Acetylcholine, 6, 7, 159-160
    action of, 161
    defined, 160
    inactivation of, 161
Actin, 166
Action potential, 12, **14-16**
    conduction velocity and, 16
    effect of
        digitalis on, 161
        diphenylhydantoin on, 164
        hyperkalemia on, 165
        hypokalemia on, 165
        lidocaine hydrochloride on, 165
        procainamide hydrochloride on, 163
        quinidine on, 163
    entrance and exit block and, 128-129
    membrane responsiveness and, 16
    of pacemaker cell, 14, 15-16
    phases of, 15-16
    reentry and, 79
    of ventricular muscle cell, 14, 15-16
Active A-V dissociation, 131-132
Active junctional rhythm defined, 90
Active rhythm defined, 51
Active ventricular extrasystoles defined, 64
Adrenalin, 158
Adrenergic defined, 158
Adrenergic drugs defined, 158
Adrenergic receptors, 157-158
    cardiovascular system and, 158
    kidneys and, 158
Alderlin; see Pronethalol
Alpha adrenergic receptors, 157-158
    blocking agents of, 159
    stimulants of, 158

Alternating current
    flow defined, 168-170
    interference, 43, 44, 180
Anterior division, left bundle branch, 102-103
Anterior wall infarct, 151
Anterobasal infarct, 151
Anterolateral infarct, 151
Anteroseptal infarct, 152-153
Antiarrhythmic drugs, 161-164
    effect on membrane responsiveness, 16
Aorta, 1, 7
Apical infarct, 152, 153
Arrest, sinus, 48
Arrhythmia
    defined, 46
    sinus, 47, **48**, 50
Arrhythmias, sinus node, 46-49
Artifacts, 42-44
Ashman's phenomenon, 108
Atria
    anatomy of, 1
    conduction velocity in, 5
    conductive system of, 5
    ECG deflection of, 35-37
    hypertrophy of, 125-126
Atrial contraction, premature, 51, **52-55**, 83, 121, 127, 131, 146, 156, 167
    bigeminal, **53**, 63
    nonconducted, 54, 55
Atrial ectopic focus, 51, 52, 55
Atrial ectopics, 51-62
Atrial fibrillation; see Fibrillation, atrial
Atrial fibrillatory line, 59
Atrial flutter; see Flutter, atrial
Atrial fusion, 136
    wandering pacemaker and, 61
Atrial hypertrophy, **125-126**, 127
Atrial standstill, 49

---

*Numbers set in boldface type indicate the principal discussion of the subject.